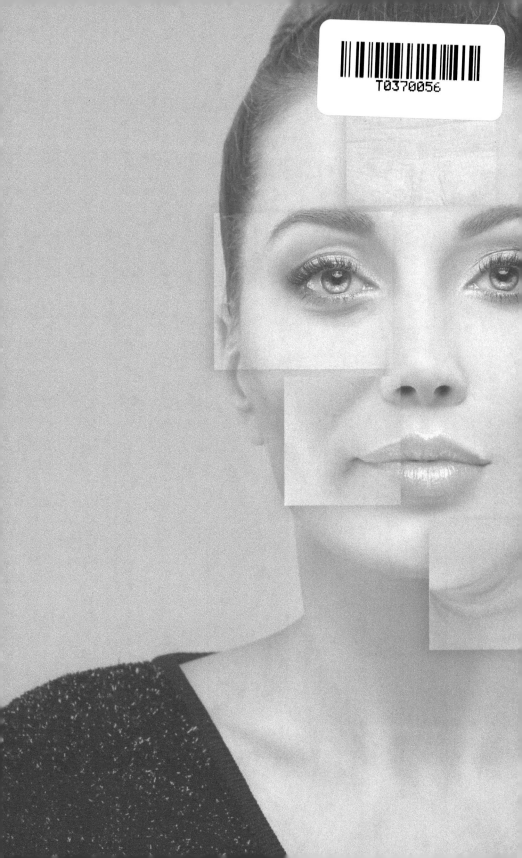

THE REAL YOU, ONLY BETTER

THE REAL YOU, ONLY BETTER

Definitive Guidance to Empower You
to Choose the Best Cosmetic Procedure
for Your Inner Beauty Transformation

**ROBERT A. HARDESTY, MD, FACS,
AND JAMES POLAKOF, PHD**

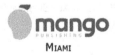

mango
PUBLISHING
MIAMI

The information provided in this book is based on the research, insights, and experiences of the author. Every effort has been made to provide accurate and up-to-date information; however, neither the author nor the publisher warrants the information provided is free of factual error. This book is not intended to diagnose, treat, or cure any medical condition or disease, nor is it intended as a substitute for professional medical care. All matters regarding your health should be supervised by a qualified healthcare professional. The author and publisher disclaim all liability for any adverse effects arising out of or relating to the use or application of the information or advice provided in this book.

For permission requests, please contact the publisher at:
Mango Publishing Group
5966 South Dixie Highway, Suite 300
Miami, FL 33143
info@mango.bz

For special orders, quantity sales, course adoptions and corporate sales, please email the publisher at sales@mango.bz. For trade and wholesale sales, please contact Ingram Publisher Services at customer.service@ingramcontent.com or +1.800.509.4887.

The Real You, Only Better: Definitive Guidance to Empower You to Choose the Best Cosmetic Procedure for Your Inner Beauty Transformation

Library of Congress Cataloging-in-Publication number: 2024941656
ISBN: (print) 978-1-68481-671-2, (ebook) 978-1-68481-672-9
BISAC category code: MED085030, MEDICAL / Surgery / Cosmetic & Reconstructive

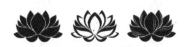

CONTENTS

PREFACE

How many have felt themselves to be prisoners in their own bodies? So often, the physical standards set forth by an imperfect society portray almost perfect physical images we must strive to abide by. In turn, this unrealistic focus stifles the very unique beauty we possess internally.

A woman who requested anonymity wrote, "For over a decade of my life, I punished my body to account for everything I thought I lacked. Believing a perfect body was the key to serenity and happiness, I became a prisoner in my own body, a slave to inhibiting my physical presence in the world. When trying to manipulate myself on the outside, I died on the inside a little more each time I gave in to self-defeating behaviors. This is how I became a prisoner in my own body."

Unlike any literary work thus far published on the subject, this book exposes the good, the bad, and the ugly of cosmetic surgery. There is a wide gap between greedy surgeons who will risk a woman's life to make a buck and those specialists who employ sensitivity and patient education to convey realistic expectations.

This book is about **empowering women to stand up for their inner beauty and not allow plastic surgery alone to define them**. And it's a "How-To" for women to access knowledge in order to best use plastic surgery as a tool to bring their real self—their inner beauty—to the surface.

It's time for both consumers interested in aesthetic procedures and plastic surgeons who perform them to reach a consensus on what true beauty actually is. We also need to recognize those lessons learned during the deadly COVID pandemic about what really matters in life. **Who we are is far more important than who we appear to be**.

Self-care has become vital to well-being. Whether it's giving yourself permission to take long bubble baths, tinkering in the backyard "she shed," enjoying herbal tea, or seeing noon come while still in your robe, being good to yourself provides a necessary reprieve from the stress and strain that life brings into our lives each day.

Additionally, as a people, we have become much more introspective. When we search inwardly, many of us discover that there is an abundance of beauty inside—far more than our physical exterior can possibly deliver.

Thus, when considering aesthetic plastic surgery, perhaps the focus should shift from glamorizing physical appearance to revealing a person's inner beauty with the help of a plastic surgeon's artistry and skill.

As authors who are knowledgeable in the aesthetic surgery field, we believe greater personal satisfaction and self-esteem can be achieved by enabling a patient's internal qualities to rise to the surface. The path toward achieving this goal is a conscious partnership between surgeon and patient to identify and capture a physical appearance which represents true inner beauty.

We believe you will find this is not another typical plastic surgery aesthetic "show and tell" book, but rather a carefully researched and well-documented literary work.

Our objective is to delve into the "why, what, and how" that any prospective consumer of cosmetic surgery procedures should consider and understand prior to choosing a surgeon and having a successful "inner beauty" outcome.

PART I

INNER BEAUTY VS. THE BEAST

Beauty and the Beast (*La Belle et la Bête*) was written by the French novelist Gabrielle-Suzanne Barbot de Villeneuve and published in 1740. The moral of the story was: "**Inner beauty is greater than physical beauty.**"

Yet plastic surgery is not a fairy tale but in fact a reality, which unfortunately is often a struggle of inner beauty repression caused by archaic, beastly attitudes and deeds. Who wins this socially induced battle is up to you!

CHAPTER 1

WHAT IS BEAUTY IN TODAY'S SOCIETY?

"The ultimate beauty that contains no contradicting elements
is beyond earthly experience."
—Socrates

One can trace debates about the essence of beauty back to the Greeks. Socrates saw beauty in its heavenly form, whereas Plato believed beauty was the object of love.

Moving forward, the Romans were quite specific about what they considered beautiful. The ideal of beauty for women was a small, thin figure with a robust constitution, narrow shoulders, pronounced hips, wide thighs, and small breasts. The canon for the face was large, almond-shaped eyes, a sharp nose, a medium-sized mouth and ears, and oval cheeks and chin. Smooth, white skin was very important for Roman women.

During the Renaissance period, women were expected to use lavish clothing, jewelry, accessories, and cosmetics to adhere to contemporary beauty standards. To be considered beautiful, a woman had to also be virtuous.

In the twentieth century, the ideals of beauty began to change with increasing speed. New concepts of feminine beauty transformed visual tastes in almost every single decade. In the 1920s, the early cinema began creating its stars. Louise Brooks and Gloria Swanson defined female beauty: small head, expressive eyes, fuller lips, and short hair were the main features.

The post-war optimism of the 1950s produced Doris Day and Debbie Reynolds, when being "sweet" was considered pretty. And then, in the 1960s, there was more concern with social protest and idealism than with feminine esthetic standards. This created a place for slender, unshapely models such as "Twiggy," who was a counterculture icon known for her thin build.

Today, what society defines as beautiful in a woman is an exaggerated hourglass: thin waist and legs, a large butt, and big breasts. (FYI: As for men, they are judged by muscle tone, shape, hairy or hairless chests, and other masculine characteristics.)

Society shapes us in many ways, possibly more than we realize—from our interactions to our personal development, to others' perception of our bodies as a reflection of self-worth.

We are social beings. Genetically, we rely on one another for the survival of humanity. That primal connection makes our interactions physiologically and psychologically important. It's not surprising that how society perceives us affects us on many levels. And it's partly how society perceives our bodies that is of concern. So what does this involve?

- How we perceive our bodies visually
- How we feel about our physical appearance
- How we think and talk to ourselves about our bodies
- Our sense of how other people view our bodies

How we look has possibly never held as much societal importance or affected so significantly our perceived self-worth. Beauty standards say that physical attractiveness is more important than a woman's other characteristics. Society in general tells so many women they are not enough, that the way they exist in this world is not beautiful, that they aren't sufficiently perfect. That's not okay.

According to *Psychology Today*, 56 percent of women say they are dissatisfied with their physical appearance, many focusing on body weight in particular. In addition, many manipulated images showcased on Instagram or Snapchat fill this insatiable void more than half of women in the modern era also find inside themselves.

It's little wonder that so many are turning to plastic surgery in hopes of becoming more compatible with today's standards of beauty. One young woman, who shall go unnamed, has a great idea:

Instead of giving in to the norm, we, as women, should put up a bigger fight against unrealistic beauty standards to empower the beauty, independence, and diversity of every individual. Taking time away from social media helps me to better combat a negative self-image. It's utterly impossible to celebrate my own unique beauty while the world feeds me a portrayal of what my physical appearance should look like.

Another lady attempting to advance a stalled career was more dramatic about her fixation with beauty. She candidly commented:

My nostrils look like bat caves. Another age spot? Why are my lips so crooked? Staring into my iPhone, I've gone from smiling to pouting to looking pensively at the camera, all to get the perfect pic for my LinkedIn profile. (I've been at this for about half an hour now.) Somewhere around the twenty-fourth shot—which, of course, I hate—I realize it's not a lighting issue or the wrong lip gloss. It's me; I'm more self-conscious and critical than ever. I don't think I was always like this.

Many women fall victim to "beauty dysmorphia." Much like body-dysmorphic disorder, a mental condition that afflicts about 2 percent of the population and makes them fixate on a perceived physical flaw that doesn't exist, beauty dysmorphia causes a warped self-image. And while it may not be a clinical diagnosis, coveting extra-pillowy lips, crease-free skin, a perfect nose, or killer cleavage (the list goes on) can cause some women to display one very real body-dysmorphic tendency: an obsession with cosmetic tweaking. And, given today's fixation with beauty, it's easier than ever to indulge in.

Oprah Winfrey has also provided meaningful advice: "Step away from the mean girls and say bye-bye to feeling bad about your looks. Are you ready to stop colluding with a culture that makes so many of us feel physically inadequate? Say goodbye to your inner critic, and take this pledge to be kinder to yourself and others."

On more than one occasion, Oprah has confessed to using food as a stress reliever. After being in the news countless times for both gaining and losing weight, Oprah has come to a point where she finally accepts her body for what it is, and she counsels others to do the same.

In today's social environment, we see ad campaigns and TV personalities that show completely unrealistic beauty standards. These expectations are detrimental to a woman's self-esteem and can push her to make questionable decisions when it comes to her own unique self.

Unrealistic beauty standards are a plague on today's society. Women look around and see expectations of what they're "supposed" to look like everywhere. This can lead to mental health issues and more. It can also cause women to try to change themselves to fit society's image.

According to the Eating Recovery Center's overview of health risks for these disorders, there is a possibility of organ damage, developmental delays, and death. Those with these disorders also have a higher chance of committing suicide. Negative body image is created by what women see around them, which can lead to succumbing to these risks. Most girls are guilty of looking in the mirror and not liking what they see. In today's society, there is a need to realize that all body types are acceptable.

Society's views of physical beauty are also affecting children. The PACEY study found that anxieties around body image are starting at a much younger age than in the past, which is why we need to have these conversations as early as possible. This is especially the case for young girls, as they are the gender most at risk for body image issues.

The Girls' Attitudes survey, which looked at 1,600 girls and young women aged seven to twenty-one, determined that the older girls get, the more ashamed they become of their appearance. If we do not teach children resilience or how to navigate body image issues, they will be more susceptible to future mental health issues such as anxiety, depression, and eating disorders.

The same holds true for adults who feel their realistic bodies and their ideal body images do not match. Several serious eating conditions are centered around body image concerns.

Those struggling with anorexia and bulimia engage in dangerous behaviors, including self-starvation, self-induced vomiting, over-exercising, and laxative abuse—all in an attempt to be in control. Oftentimes, their image and weight are the only things they have control over, since they are continuously repressed by underlying depression or anxiety.

Beauty Can Have a Negative Impact on Women's Careers

An interesting article in *Forbes* magazine revealed findings from a recent study. "Good-looking people are not only regarded as more physically attractive; they are also generally credited with having more positive personalities. But researchers have shown that this is not the case for beautiful women in professional life, especially when it comes to securing managerial positions with major organizations."

Women seeking management positions with major organizations may consider this good news—and it is. However, more recently, researchers at Yale University made an important discovery. Per the article:

> These researchers designed and conducted an experiment to test the hypothesis that physical attractiveness is always an advantage in a business environment. They presented their test subjects with job applications from equivalently qualified applicants—but with very different photos attached to each application. One-half included portrait photographs of attractive applicants; the other half had pictures of unattractive applicants. Apart from this, there was no difference between the applications or applicants.

However, the researchers did add a variable to their experiment: They depicted the first job as an average-paying position at level eight in the twenty-one-level hierarchy of a large company. The second was a very well-paid decision-making position at level sixteen in the hierarchy.

The result was certainly interesting. For male applicants, good looks were a definite advantage when it came to the managerial job: 43.5 percent of test subjects thought that the more attractive male candidate was better suited for the top position, while only 13 percent said the same about the unattractive male applicant. The opposite was true for women:

30.5 percent of subjects awarded the unattractive female candidate the highest ranking for the managerial job, while only 13 percent chose the attractive female applicant.

The situation was completely reversed when it came to applications for the nonmanagerial job. In this case, 47 percent of subjects preferred the more attractive female candidate, in contrast to the 16 percent who chose the less-attractive applicant.

The key finding:

> These data strongly suggest that whether attractiveness is a help or a hindrance to job applicants depends upon the sex of the applicant and the nature of the job he or she seeks. Whereas attractiveness consistently proved to provide an advantage for male applicants seeking white-collar organizational positions, it was an advantage for female applicants only when the position was a nonmanagerial one.

Thus, according to the researchers, there is a distinct tendency for attractiveness to work *against* female applicants for managerial positions. The researchers assumed that this discrimination was based on the fact that managerial positions are associated with "masculine" gender attributes—and the more feminine attributes a woman is considered to have, the less suitable she appears for a top job.

As a result, the researchers recommended that career-oriented women should be aware of the potency of first impressions during the application process: "This finding sadly implies that women should strive to appear as unattractive and as masculine as possible if they are to succeed in advancing their careers by moving into powerful organizational positions."

Recent Study: Attractive Women Tend to Be Mistrusted

A recent university study, conducted by Professor Leah D. Sheppard and Professor Stefanie K. Johnson and published by Harvard Business Publishing in 2019, concluded that for women in business, beauty is a liability. However, these researchers posited different reasons to explain the negative impact of attractiveness on women's careers. They conducted six experiments to test whether people are predisposed to trust highly attractive rather than less-attractive female company leaders when they announce positive or negative organizational news. But no matter what the news was, the female beauty penalty persisted.

The female researchers called this the "femme fatale effect." Through variants of their experiment, they attempted to prove that previous efforts to explain discrimination against beautiful women as the result of the stereotype that women are not considered a good "fit" for "masculine" management positions were not convincing. Employing a series of different experiments, they then sought to demonstrate that the real reason for such discrimination was "that attractive women could often elicit sexual jealousy among those who regard them, even in the context of the workplace, which could then have negative implications for their perceived truthfulness and trustworthiness." This could, they suggest, fuel suspicions that a beautiful woman could use her sexual attractiveness to gain career advantages that are not based on her performance.

Why Attractive People Are More Successful in Life

Regardless of recent individual studies, there is an overall consensus that attractive individuals generally enjoy greater success. The preponderance of research reveals you're more likely to get hired if you look well-groomed, that good-looking people make about 12 percent more money than less physically appealing folks, and attractive candidates are more likely to get elected. Psychologists call it the "beauty premium."

The only way this is going to change is if society begins to open up to different types of beauty besides the expected ones. All races, body shapes, hairstyles, and stretch marks should be socially acceptable. Moving forward and away from the outdated beauty standards is essential. Doing this will give all women the confidence they need to be themselves without fear of judgment. It is now time for more social leaders to speak out, emphasizing that the real beauty of a person goes beyond physical appearance.

In a humorous but honest evaluation, Tina Fey calls out society for its ridiculous physical standards for women:

> Now every girl is expected to have Caucasian blue eyes, full Spanish lips, a classic button nose, hairless Asian skin with a Californian tan, a Jamaican dance hall ass, long Swedish legs, small Japanese feet, the abs of a lesbian gym owner, the hips of a nine-year-old boy, the arms of Michelle Obama, and doll tits. The person closest to actually achieving this look is Kim Kardashian, who, as we know, was made by Russian scientists to sabotage our athletes.

On a more serious note, Taylor Swift provides a more realistic expectation: "I definitely have body issues, but everybody does. When you come to the realization that everybody does—even the people that I consider flawless—then you can start to live with the way you are."

Dr. Hardesty: As a plastic surgeon, I believe we should pay less attention to society's misguided standards of beauty and focus more on a person's feeling about what makes them beautiful. Defining beauty is individualistic and highly subjective. In my daily professional life, I have been struck by the wide variation of patient desires. Here are two examples.

Some women who have genetically large breasts complain that "size" limits their ability to exercise, or they experience physical ailments such as neck and back pain because of the weight of their breasts. Thus, they request that I perform a breast reduction.

Conversely, certain women are fortunate to be born with nicely shaped but smaller breasts, and now feel self-conscious due to a perception of inadequate size.

In the first example, restriction and pain are excellent reasons for surgical intervention. As for the second case, my policy is to recommend to those patients that their decision with regard to surgery should be based upon their personal aspirations, and not an image that society advocates.

Dr. Polakof: Readers may be curious why our focus upon beauty is largely female-oriented, as opposed to targeting men as well. The fact is, women represent 90 percent of all aesthetic plastic surgery procedures, and society's beauty mores tend to cause greater harm to the female population.

Numerous studies verify that the feminine beauty ideal is a socially constructed opinion that one of a woman's most important assets is attractiveness—something all women should attempt to attain. Suntanned skin, a narrower facial shape, high cheekbones, longer eyelashes, fuller lips, and a curvaceous body are just a few of the qualities that are considered attractive for women in modern Western society.

Whether women are conscious of it or not, most are striving to attain the beauty ideals that society perpetuates and encourages.

Additionally, women have long been the primary target of many marketers, not just because they make up roughly half of the entire world's population, but because of their sheer buying power. Reports vary, but it's believed women drive 70 to 80 percent of all consumer purchasing decisions.

As a result, major companies stress the stereotypes of attractiveness for women to motivate purchasing. Just as many plastic surgeons need to refocus upon capturing a woman's inner beauty, companies must realize that a new day is dawning in their traditional marketplace.

CHAPTER 2

WHAT IS INNER BEAUTY?

The Roles of Sex & Career

"People often say that 'beauty is in the eye of the beholder,' and I say that the most liberating thing about beauty is realizing that you are the beholder. This empowers us to find beauty in places where others have not dared to look, including inside ourselves."

—Salma Hayek

What makes attractive people so attractive? You may think it's a chiseled face or a gorgeous physique that makes a person attractive. But more than anything else, it's a person's inner belief that they're attractive that makes them more appealing to others.

You don't choose someone to be part of your life because of how pretty or tall they are. You select the person because of their kindness, wisdom, or generosity—all of which are part of inner beauty.

The glow of confidence and sex appeal comes from within yourself. You're confident because of how you present yourself to the world and because you maintain your authenticity. Many people assume that confidence has everything to do with your physical appearance, but that's not true. Some of the most fancied personalities, like Oprah, Lady Gaga, or Tom Hanks, aren't necessarily the prettiest of people in the conventional sense. But their glowing confidence and self-belief make them attractive to every member of the opposite sex.

Society has led us to believe that everyone will judge us based on our physical appearance. However, first impressions don't always depend on your physique, but you need to believe that from within yourself. And that's where your true beauty lies. More than what you look like, your true worth lies within.

Are You Beautiful on the Inside?

Inner beauty helps you appreciate outer beauty. If you feel good about yourself, you will feel more confident about facing and interacting with other individuals. Even if outer beauty is tangible, it's not enough to make someone stay in your life.

The factor that really makes you attractive is your capacity to use your heart and values when it matters. People are more attracted to you when you speak up with courage or when you act in a selfless way. Remember, outer beauty can win you a glance, but it's inner beauty that makes someone stay.

Even when you look at an inanimate object, like a painting or a spectacular view of the ocean, it seems more beautiful to you because you see the beauty that overflows within you reflected in everything else around you. And that's when you'll realize that the ability to see beauty comes from within yourself.

If you tend to see the glass as half empty, this could also reflect your inability to see beauty in people and things around you. If you perceive yourself as lacking inner beauty, then that perspective can reflect on everyone you cross paths with. If you truly felt beautiful on the inside, you'd never seem unappealing to anyone else.

The real definition of beauty should be focused on what makes a person their most authentic self, regardless of whether this refers to their looks or their characteristics. You're beautiful if you believe you're beautiful. You're attractive if you feel attractive. Everyone only sees you as a projection of what you see when you look into the mirror.

The Story of a Woman in Her Forties

Barrie is a teacher now in her late forties. Recently, her children were just about out of the nest. She was beginning to once again feel young and carefree, starting to laugh again and feel silly with her friends. That was until she took a close look at herself in a mirror. According to Barrie, "Suddenly, my own distorted self-perceptions around aging and appearance quickly brought me back to the reality of who I was on the outside and how I was supposed to behave." She goes on to tell an all-too-familiar story:

> I'd previously stared in the mirror many times, pulling the skin back on my face to see how many years a facelift might remove. But this was the first time I realized the subtle toll my self-perceptions were taking on my psyche and self-confidence.
>
> Somewhere inside of me, I believed middle-aged women didn't sing and laugh and act silly. That was reserved for the young and beautiful. In our youth- and beauty-obsessed culture, every time we open a magazine, turn on the TV, or drive past a billboard, we

see how far our personal reality is from the standard perpetuated by the media. These messages were obviously entrenched in me, but I didn't truly wake up to it until I applied the harsh judgment to myself.

Was I really going to allow these messages to keep me from feeling beautiful and carefree? And more importantly, as my physical appearance continues to change, is my self-worth going to diminish more and more over time because society tells me I'm no longer relevant?

These images and messages don't just affect those pushing forty or beyond. Young women in today's culture see more images of exceptionally beautiful women in one day than our mothers saw throughout their entire teenage years. It's no wonder that eight out of ten women are dissatisfied with their appearance.

By any chance, do you recognize this story? Sadly, the statistic is fairly accurate, but still, it's hard to believe that so many women have such a negative view of their appearance. It was then that Barrie decided to reverse her fortunes and not settle for this age-old stigma.

Barrie continues:

What if true beauty were defined by who we are rather than how we look? What if it was okay to have flaws, to be less-than-perfect—not only okay but actually preferred and even celebrated?

This was a huge shift for me that has led to self-acceptance. Yes, there are some elements of our faces and bodies we simply cannot change. Rather than resisting and struggling against these things, relax into them and accept them with love.

Struggle and resistance do nothing but push us further away from recognizing our true beauty. Acknowledge and accept those parts of your appearance you have grown to hate. View them as children who long for and deserve your love and acceptance.

As I've grown older, I've consciously redirected my focus away from dwelling on my appearance. Yes, I still do what I can to look attractive and presentable. I exercise and eat a healthy diet. But I try not to obsess about the changes my face and body are undergoing.

I recognize that my true beauty shines from expressing my authentic self, from the joy I experience in daily life, and from my interactions with loving friends and family. For me, true beauty comes from living fully, being who I am, and experiencing the beauty all around me.

When you find yourself doubting your own true beauty, please remember, as Khalil Gibran so eloquently reminds us, "Beauty is not in the face; beauty is a light in the heart."

I say, allow the light in your heart to shine for yourself and others, and in so doing, your entire being will glow with a fire of beauty. You will be a beacon of attractiveness to everyone you encounter.

Excellent advice. Thank you, Barrie!

Outer Beauty Will Never Compare to the Depth That Inner Beauty Can Provide

It focuses on everything regarding your physical appearance. No matter how much effort you put into your makeup or the clothes you wear, it's not going to get you more than a second glance. Outer beauty might give others the first impression that they need you, but inner beauty reflects your worth more.

The following are advantages that provide an understanding as to why inner beauty is more important:

- Inner beauty doesn't have an expiration date, unlike external beauty, which biologically wanes with age.

- Inner beauty is the strength in relationships, while an external appearance does not create lasting bonds.

People with inner beauty are well-connected to their emotions. They are, therefore, better decision-makers and thinkers.

- Inner beauty gives you the confidence to face the world and its problems, which is something far greater than the standards that have been set by society.

- Inner beauty is unlikely to be judged. While judgment is a constant companion of external appearance, inner beauty most often receives praise.

Developing your inner beauty will also give you your own sense of self-worth and help your body in achieving harmony and proper functioning with its bodily systems. Amazing health benefits can be experienced by a person who truly works on all aspects of their inner beauty.

A Woman's Inner Beauty

Inner beauty consists of those stunning and attractive traits in a woman that are above and beyond her physical attractiveness. A woman may be gorgeous outside and have a great inner beauty, while others may be gorgeous on the outside and ugly on the inside. We also have other women who don't fit society's standards of being beautiful but have both inner and outer beauty.

Inner beauty makes a woman more attractive, since it relies more on personality and behaviors toward other people. She may possess such traits as kindness, charity, and selflessness. The inner beauty of a woman shines through other people and her actions toward others, and it cannot be faked; it's natural, eliciting sincere and genuine responses.

True beauty is hard to define, but it involves the characteristics of a person that provide perceptual experiences of satisfaction, meaning, and pleasure. The most common qualities of inner beauty include tenderness, sensitivity, creativity, compassion, intelligence, and kindness. Here are the top characteristics of a woman's inner beauty:

- Developing your spiritual nature
- Being yourself
- Being confident
- Avoiding revenge and jealousy
- Exercising regularly
- Being humble
- Caring about the environment
- Caring for the less fortunate
- Being disciplined
- Having the power to control emotions
- Not diminishing others
- Keeping on smiling

Inner beauty is always the real beauty. Looks are deceptive, while the traits of a person reveal their internal thinking. Having admirable character brings out your inner beauty, and speaking to other people with respect brings out a unique style that is attractive.

A woman with inner beauty is vulnerable, and yet she is self-assured, possessing ethical and noble manners with the energy of softness, mystery, cleverness, and strength.

The Role Sex Plays in Inner Beauty

Psychologists contend that **possessing a healthy attitude about your sexuality will help you bring out your inner beauty.** In an article for Self.com, counselor/therapist Teresa Maples-Zuvela writes:

Experts say, "A sexually healthy person is someone who feels comfortable with her or his sexuality." This means, a person doesn't view sex as something naughty, bad, improper, or sinful and can engage in it without feeling guilty or anxious. When you're comfortable with who you are on the inside, your attractiveness is infectious on the outside. Others want to be around you and have what you have. The movie *Shallow Hal* is a good example of physically portraying a woman's inner beauty. Hal only dated women who were physically beautiful. One day, however, he gets hypnotized to recognize only the inner beauty of women. Hal then meets a grossly obese woman and all he can see is her inner beauty. Beauty from within comes from feeling good about you.

Sure, attraction matters. Love is not blind. However, spend enough time with someone, and you'll realize that looks are just an appetizer, a small, unstable frame in the architecture of happiness. Even a perfect diamond will crack with bad chemistry.

Outer beauty is simple. You see it. You get it. Inner beauty has many shades and colors. You have to explore to find them. But, upon discovery, they're yours. They don't fade. You can savor them forever.

Sapiosexuality

By definition, a sapiosexual is someone who finds intelligence sexually attractive or arousing—and this has become an emerging trend. The word "sapiosexual" originated from the Latin root word *sapien*, which means wise, and *sexualis*, which means sexual.

Because sapiosexuals are attracted to intellect, they can't be attracted without the brain being triggered. There is no lust, liking, wanting, or sexual gratification unless the brain has been stimulated on an intellectual level first.

Since they value intelligence more than looks, sapiosexuals show their attraction for others in a way that's different from the norm. So if a sapiosexual is interested in you romantically, you can be sure that they value you for more than the way you look.

How do you know if you're a sapiosexual? You prefer deep conversations, you require intellect in a potential partner, and you believe intelligence is sexier than a "beach bod."

How Do Men View the Beauty of Women?

While there is something to the notion that men judge beauty because it's what they see, times are changing!

In fact, we find the stereotyped viewpoint of many men is evolving in a positive direction. As an example, here is the statement of a man from Texas during an interview:

> What I find funny is that the things that girls don't like [about themselves], I end up enjoying. Such as the way she could laugh

or if her nose crinkles a bit when she is focusing on something. For me personally, the little things that a girl may dislike about herself, I end up loving. If a perfect God made man (and woman of course) in his image, then how can a lady think she is anything less than perfect? Yes, we may have earthly eyes, but we can always change our perspective.

It breaks my heart when women view themselves as less. Less of anything really because the truth is that they are so much more but are letting the things around them limit them. It is super cliché but the biggest limiting factor we have is our mind. I know it is not easy for a girl to just believe she is pretty or loved or worthy or wanted, but like most good things, it takes time. Also, it's just a truth that one broken person will not feel whole with someone by their side. One thing (that I do not tell the girls I date too often) that I absolutely love is staring at her. When she is not looking and we are lying down on a couch or something, I love looking at every single intricate twist and turn and freckle. I find that beautiful. It is unique to her.

And here is a comment made by a man from Arizona: "I appreciate women when they show their nurturing side. I just think it's beautiful when their feminine qualities shine through."

Let's not leave out a New Mexico gentleman: "Personally, I like that women can be independent and find it beautiful when they aren't afraid to show their intellectualism."

And finally, a man from Pennsylvania:

It's hard for me to name a characteristic I appreciate "generically" in women because all the women I know are incredibly diverse and all of them have different but amazing talents and personality traits. I've become good friends with very outgoing women, very quiet women, very artistic women, women who are amazingly gifted in STEM fields, women who have sacrificed everything for their families, and women who have devoted their lives to the pursuit of a noble ambition. And I wouldn't consider any of these women to be "more feminine" or "less feminine" than any other woman. I don't know how much of a right I have to say this as a guy, but I think femininity has nothing to do with wearing expensive makeup or clothes, or the number of hours you spend styling your hair. It has everything to do with accepting the beautiful and immeasurably precious existence that you already are and never allowing your soul to be shut into the Barbie doll box the world tells you it should be in.

Dr. Hardesty: The real definition of "total beauty," I believe, should include and focus on what makes a person their most genuine authentic self. I strongly believe we are only as beautiful as we believe we are. First impressions are important, but are only a segue to understanding the true "total" beauty of a person. Inner beauty is the real and true beauty of a person that amplifies the external and goes far beyond just physical appearances. Inner beauty, at first glance, might not be seen, but it goes far beyond what the eye sees and the hand touches.

Dr. Polakof: Inner beauty is spiritual in the sense that it has the ability to touch the soul and make it feel joyful. There is a simple and yet deep impact it can have on any person. It is so subtle that we often tend to forget the significance of having and cultivating inner beauty. We often forget it is the warmth and the love we give to and receive from other people that makes it possible for us to feel the attachments and enrichment.

Inner beauty is something that will last forever. It has the ability to make people love you no matter what. The kind of love and appreciation that is true, deep, and real. Nourish your inner beauty to enable it to blossom and grow deeper with expanding joy!

> "Why try to be an attractive oyster when you can be the precious pearl inside it?"
> —Anonymous

CHAPTER 3

BE THE QUEEN OF YOUR HEART

Protect and Project Your Beauty

"People always ask me, 'You have so much confidence. Where did that come from?' It came from me. One day I decided that I was beautiful, and so I carried out my life as if I was a beautiful girl. It doesn't have anything to do with how the world perceives you. What matters is what you see. Your body is your temple. It's your home, and you must decorate it."

—Gabourey Sidibe

What does it mean to be "you"—that is, to have a specific, conscious experience of the world around you and yourself within it? There may be no more elusive or fascinating question. Historically, humanity has considered the nature of consciousness to be a primarily spiritual or philosophical inquiry, but scientific research is now mapping out compelling biological theories and explanations for consciousness and selfhood.

Neuroscience to the rescue! As a window into your consciousness of being "you," consider that we do not perceive the world as it objectively is, but rather that we are prediction machines, constantly inventing our world and correcting our mistakes by the microsecond, and that we can now observe the biological mechanisms in the brain that accomplish this process of consciousness.

Have you ever admired someone and pondered how they've achieved such inner beauty? It's certainly not about outward appearance. Instead, this person exudes positive qualities that make them a genuinely beautiful soul.

By now you may have guessed it. The concept of beauty isn't limited to having high cheekbones, whopper boobs, or, more recently, that perfect thigh gap. If you come to know and love the entirety of yourself, your body, mind, and soul, the outside beauty becomes less relevant, and a different kind of attractiveness overshadows the rest.

You need to learn to take care of yourself first before you can take care of others. It is often difficult for women to set boundaries and put their needs first when they are in a relationship. Just like a passenger on an airplane, you will be better equipped to take care of others if you put your own oxygen mask on first.

Taking care of yourself includes making your mental and physical health a priority, as well as learning how to set healthy boundaries and how to say a loving "no." Boundaries will always lead to healthier relationships and social interactions. Here are considerations to help guide you in this direction:

You Are More Than Your Looks

Discover your uniqueness and own it! Knowing yourself, your beliefs, what matters most to you, and what "goodness" is in you are the important steps in identifying your inner beauty. This is where positive thinking kicks in and confidence can reign supreme!

Inner Detox—Redirect Negative Thoughts

There are times when we can't help but feel bombarded by negative thoughts. They can arise from feelings such as wanting an hourglass figure, perky breasts, a nice jawline, or to get rid of increasing wrinkles. Such thoughts can take an immense toll on how we feel about ourselves. Of course, you can make improvements with plastic surgery—and why not? But first, you need to remind yourself that these are only minor deficiencies and are far less important than the inner beauty you possess.

Create Boundaries to Protect You in Life's Geographic Pitfalls

Remove anyone or anything that doesn't bring joy or happiness to your life. The energy you let in is crucial and can impact you without you even noticing. It can either bring you down or lift you up. Preserve your space and focus on being around people who want to see you shine and bring out the absolute best in you.

Don't Get Caught up in Social Media

We are all aware of how destructive social media has been to the lives of many. It often tempts us to compare ourselves with others or become upset by insensitive comments from fair-weather friends. Social media can sometimes become a black hole that sucks you in, so be aware of when you need to take a break and unplug. Always strive to shut off the negative and focus upon the positive—which is your inner beauty!

Plastic Surgery Can Be Your Friend

If you can truly recognize your inner beauty and not become obsessed with minor physical imperfections, plastic surgery can then enhance the confidence you already possess. If there is a physical feature that has bothered you for a long period of time, that interferes with looking as good as you feel, then spend time to research a good surgeon and take advantage of safe procedures that can help. Dealing with an issue you have with your physical self can actually help you feel more beautiful on the inside. But don't hold things inside. It's important that you communicate your inner beauty qualities to a sensitive plastic surgeon. He or she can then help you better achieve your objectives.

Be the Queen of Your Heart

Discovering your inner beauty means you need to be the "queen of your own heart." Being the "queen of your own heart" takes a lot of work and means you have to look deep inside in the darkest places so that you can take authority over them. Just as a queen would do, seek counsel on how to overcome the pain. Do not retreat from the pain, but face it head-on and look at it in an objective manner so that it has no influence over you. Take a look back at those difficult moments and times when you have felt less than yourself and think of how you allowed those times to define you.

Do not crumble at the raising of another's sharp sword. Instead, stand strong and ask yourself in every negative situation, "Is this going to define me? What am I going to receive from it?" It's our job to understand the implications of our heart story and what we choose to be true of us. Ask yourself, "What healing of the heart do I need to do in order to receive the truth of my heart?" It is only when we clear away the lies and see ourselves for who we are that we are able to be the queen who reigns with a beauty that may not be seen, but can be felt. This is the definition of internal beauty.

You Are Not Your Body

You've heard the phrase "heart and soul"—in fact, it was a song that originated in 1938. The bottom line is that you are not your body...you are your "heart." It's what's inside that really counts. That's how the world should work. Sadly, we let comments on appearance dominate our conversations and our priorities. Hearing someone say your personality matters more than how good your hair looks that day isn't always believable when compliments tend to be outwardly focused. We live in a world that tells us inner beauty counts but does everything to contradict it.

Inner beauty really does count, but oftentimes it doesn't change what you see in the mirror or ease the pain that comes from feeling "less than" the people around you.

When someone tells you that your heart and mind matter most, of course you want to believe it. You also want to trust that you're seen as a beautiful person because of the way you love people, or love life, but it can be difficult to get to that state of mind.

The value of inner beauty gets overlooked when we leave it out of our daily conversations. So, instead of approaching someone and immediately jumping into a conversation about their outfit, start with something deeper. Make what's inside count. It isn't going to happen unless you are intentional about it. You decide where conversations lead. If you're only approaching others about their outer beauty, don't be surprised when they can't see the attractiveness of your inner beauty.

It's truly up to us to change this reality. The beauty of someone's heart should be one of the first things we fall in love with, but you can't properly appreciate someone's heart if you don't take the time to hear about what's in it.

Ask people what they value. Ask about what is exciting or challenging in their life. Go further than compliments by approaching a conversation with questions that express interest. This means going beyond, "How are you?" and being purposeful and enthusiastic about knowing people deeply. Make it a priority to listen to people talk about their hopes and dreams.

It's certainly not out of line to compliment people, but express that you "see" how beautiful they are. This will cause most individuals to take a deeper look inside you. It's important to find a good balance between complimenting outer beauty and being intentional about acknowledging inner beauty.

Ralph Waldo Emerson said:

> To laugh often and much; to win the respect of intelligent people and the affection of children; to earn the appreciation of honest critics and endure the betrayal of false friends; to appreciate beauty, to find the best in others; to leave the world a bit better, whether by a healthy child, a garden patch, or a redeemed social condition; to know even one life has breathed easier because you have lived. This is to have succeeded.

While Emerson does not specifically expand upon it, his quotation embodies many qualities of inner beauty. He talks about appreciating beauty while finding the best in others, which is exactly the balance we should have.

The Understated Qualities of a Beautiful Woman

As we have discussed, there is currently too great a value assigned to external beauty. For some people, how they look physically may simply be an expression and celebration of their internal beauty, but often those who are physically attractive are emotionally unattractive. To be beautiful inside and out, you must possess more than a pretty shell. Thus, let's examine those qualities individuals possess that may be under-emphasized.

Graceful Elegance: Elegance is that dignified grace about your appearance, movement, personal style, or behavior. To be elegant is to be strong and assured in who you are and to move gently within that energy. When you possess elegance, you are graceful even amidst a challenge. You are able to handle yourself in a noble and ethical manner. You hold good posture; your energy has a mystery, softness, strength, and cleverness to it. You are vulnerable yet self-assured. Elegance is the undeniable quality of the depth of your personal wisdom.

Kindness: The kindness of your spirit—how you treat, think about, and speak to others—comes from a genuine and sensitive place. You are kind, even to those whom you may not care for.

Being kind may be perceived as weakness or vulnerability by others, but you know that kindness is one of your strongest virtues. If you can't say something nice, you have the control to remain quiet. There is no human quality that will get you further in life than kindness.

Self-Control: Composure is the beauty of self-control. Life is always going to bring its challenges. Without a sense of composure, it is easy to allow conflictual situations and relationships to unnerve you, but when you have composure, you understand the concept of "less equals more."

The less you react, defend, explain, and become fearful or controlling, the more command you have over a situation. Having composure allows you to stand tall with grace in the face of loss or challenge and not be overly boastful when it comes to your success.

Confidence: When you are self-loving, you naturally possess a quiet confidence. Your self-awareness, dedication to self-development, and personal growth provide you the knowledge to succeed at nearly anything you seek.

Because of your life experiences and inner depth, you can be certain positive things will happen in your life because you depend upon yourself to have the information and willingness to do the work necessary to get to your result.

Your Identity: You are clear and persistent about who you are, where you are headed in life, and what you want from your relationships to be happy. Because you are deliberate, people know where they stand with you. You get what you want in life because you are clear in stating what you want.

You use each challenge life brings to further refine yourself. This refinement keeps your life clean of negativity. Being deliberate keeps you pointed in the direction of your dreams, connected to your true loves, and living genuinely as who you are. In being deliberate, your life is not set up on pretenses. Who you are does not change from person to person or situation to situation.

Be Courageous: Be willing to dare greatly in your life. It takes courage to love fully, to change yourself when necessary, to feel deeply, to leave love when it's scary, and to chase your dreams with passion and an unwavering tenacity.

You are aware that to become courageous you must do courageous things. You also know it is not the loudness of your mouth but the depth of your character that makes you thrive, no matter your circumstances.

Intelligence: Intelligence is about knowledge, but even more so about emotions. In being aware of your emotional patterns, you are endowed with the flexibility to handle challenge and change, allowing you to unlock smart solutions to your problems.

With a well-rounded intelligence, you carry yourself in a stately and unafraid manner. You are secure knowing there are a multitude of choices available in life, so there is no need to be reactive. In being emotionally intelligent, you have the ability to keep your eyes on the bigger picture, turning obstacles into opportunities.

Humility: Life isn't all about you; in fact, you prefer to celebrate the accomplishments of others as much as your own. You are proud of who you are, but have no need to add theatrics to your success. Most of the time, you prefer being in the background, working hard and allowing your success to speak for itself.

You are sensitive and want the best for everyone. You do not see yourself as above others, as you are secure enough in yourself that the trap of comparison doesn't interest you. You enjoy your life for what it is and do not feel entitled to more without the commensurate work to back it up.

Honesty: People gravitate toward what is real. You are simple, up-front, gentle, but direct in the "being" of who you are. You are content to live life patiently, and you know how to wait well. For you, life is about being authentic and following your heart and nothing else. You are someone others can depend upon, as you have no ulterior motives.

You are relationship-oriented, not agenda-oriented. You believe the truth is the only path to success and deep intimacy. You do not change who you are based on who you are with. You are who you are, and your priority in life is to feel happy and satisfied.

Loving: There is nothing more appealing to others than to be in the presence of a loving person. When you love yourself, you have endless love to give. For you, love is a verb, and it expresses itself through loving kindness, touch, your smile, and a sense of inner joy and vitality.

You are warm toward others and kind to yourself. There is nothing you wouldn't do to help, and this loving approach is taken into every area of your life, from career to parenting. Furthermore, you apply love as a form of discipline and set boundaries when necessary.

There are times when the only way another can learn and grow is for you to either withdraw your love or set boundaries around it in an effort to protect your generous nature. You know that, in order for you to remain loving, you must protect your heart and not put yourself in negative situations. Through life's experiences, you have come to accept that some people can stay in your heart but not in your life.

To be truly beautiful, it is the understated qualities of beauty that are sustaining. To possess any one of them will increase the experience of your beauty exponentially. Who you are internally is the marker of your influence on the world.

Gorgeous Georgia—A Story of Inner Beauty

Gorgeous Georgia is a giraffe and...well...she's just plain gorgeous! Georgia knows it and feels inclined to tell everyone so. She brags about her lovely, long neck, beautiful chestnut brown spots, graceful, lengthy legs, and her long, blue tongue.

The other animals find her objectionable. Georgia has the misconception of thinking that telling all the other animals in the forest about her beauty will make them naturally want to know her. Instead, due to her boastful and abrasive personality, they stay away from her. Georgia is left feeling lonely. As a defense mechanism, she finds herself making fun of the other animals.

As her morning ritual, Georgia stares at her gorgeous reflection in the lake. One fateful day, she slips and scrapes her neck on a branch that will leave an inevitable scar down the length of her lovely neck. The other animals feel no desire to help her.

Until...Sabra, the wise old lioness, tells them the sad story of Georgia's childhood, which was filled with loneliness. Her parents were taken to the zoo, and she was left on her own. The animals begin to feel compassion for Georgia and understand her need to feel liked. They rescue her from the lake. They start noticing and enjoying her good traits.

The moral of this story is that Georgia learns that inner beauty is far greater than superficial outside looks, and that to have friends, you must be a friend. The other animals have also learned a lesson: Do not judge others before understanding their circumstances.

Dr. Hardesty: It's a fact that aesthetic plastic surgery can help to improve self-confidence and make you feel better about yourself. But before choosing surgery, you should know that you are doing it for yourself only. Make sure you know what you really want to achieve with your procedure. Talk to your plastic surgeon to have a better understanding of what your results may look like, and how you may feel after the procedure is complete. A trustworthy and talented surgeon can help you boost your confidence and improve your appearance.

Dr. Polakof: Of course, undergoing plastic surgery to make our noses smaller or our stomachs flatter can make us feel more confident in our bodies. However, it is not realistic for us to think that plastic surgery will instantly make us feel great and no longer have low self-esteem. Improving self-esteem is a feat that will take more than just plastic surgery to achieve, since, as we have learned, there are many factors involved. That being said, in some cases, plastic surgery can definitely help you get there and might just be a positive step in your overall journey.

CHAPTER 4

GOOD REASONS FOR PLASTIC SURGERY

"No one can or should tell you why you should consider plastic surgery for aesthetic reasons. You should be able to clearly define your desire to improve aging or enhance facial or body appearance. Others may support you in your decision, but the decision to have plastic surgery should be yours alone."

—Diane Gerber

There is no doubt that aesthetic plastic surgery procedures can change your life. In the modern world, there has been a significant social shift in the way people view plastic surgery. There has been an increase in available information and discussion.

Even celebrities and media personalities have begun to speak more openly about their surgical procedures, freely discussing their cosmetic journeys on social media outlets.

Many more people are now of the view that there is certainly nothing wrong with helping nature along. In fact, we all do this in various other ways, be they surgical or cosmetic. If you care about your appearance and want to maintain a balanced body or youthful features, then there is also nothing wrong with wanting to reduce the visible signs of aging.

However, there can occasionally be negative opinions and discussions about people who choose to change their appearance through aesthetic plastic surgery. This can be due to closed thinking and concerns regarding the impact of photoshopped media images and the effect it can have on body image—as well as the effect it can have on the younger generation.

Body image and the psychological problems involved should certainly be taken seriously, although such complex issues have and will continue to exist regardless of plastic surgery. The most important consideration is that enhancing your appearance should not be done to impress others but to please yourself.

Plastic surgery can be a positive, life-changing experience. Effective plastic surgery can build confidence and eliminate a person's self-conscious thoughts on typical body concerns. It may not have a dramatic life-changing effect, but aesthetic plastic surgery can bring a level of confidence to one's appearance which resonates within daily life.

A patient who wished to share her story explained her surgical decision in the following way:

> I've had plastic surgery for reasons other than medical necessity. I did it because my body had flaws I just couldn't accept, and there was an option available to change it. Because of my conflicting—or shameful—feelings about cosmetic surgery, I feel the need to further explain my rationale.
>
> I lost more than three hundred pounds after a gastric bypass and had a *lot* of excess skin. I had very pronounced chest tissue that

made me look—and feel—terrible. I do admit that I like the way I look now better than before.

The potential adverse psychological and social effects of plastic surgery have a lot to do with a patient's preoperative expectations and their preoperative mental and emotional state. It's important to understand that, while plastic surgery can bring positive rewards, it will not change your life, the problems you have, or issues in your relationships. It is also important to understand that there is no such thing as physical "perfection."

For many patients, successful plastic surgery can lead to an increase in self-esteem and confidence. Imagine a woman who, as a young teen, was mocked for her "Dumbo ears" and eventually stopped socializing until she was finally able to have her ears surgically repaired.

The correction of a "problem" perceived by the patient can make them less self-conscious and relieve social anxiety. It may make them more outgoing, less vulnerable, and more willing to show off their new, flattering features. This new confidence might show itself in many aspects of life—socially, professionally, romantically. When you feel comfortable and confident in your own skin, you will radiate these positive emotions in everything you do.

While social pressure plays a role in influencing the felt need for such procedures, personal satisfaction is a far greater motivator than vanity. The enhancement of self-esteem and confidence provides an excellent reason.

Health and Quality of Life

In some cases, plastic surgery can yield distinct improvements in quality of life. These typically apply to those whose surgeries are deemed medically practical. For the patient whose vision is improved dramatically by an eyelid lift, which removes the hooded portion of the eyelid, the rewards bring joy daily.

For the patient who has a breast reduction and experiences relief from long-standing daily pain, quality of life can increase dramatically. For the patient who has twenty pounds of loose hanging skin after weight loss removed from their body, it can mean feeling comfortable with increased levels of physical activity.

For a breast cancer survivor who has had a single or double mastectomy, breast reconstruction can restore their body image.

For a patient who has lived with an obviously visible disfigurement, reconstructive surgery can make that person feel free again—able to face a world that is no longer staring—and live free from the judgment they experienced before. In many cases, plastic surgery can be a tremendous life-changing event.

Meet Women Who Describe Their Reasons for Plastic Surgery and Results

Amy was a fifty-four-year-old mother and grandmother who began noticing her face and neck had taken a turn for the worse in her eyes. She'd developed jowls, and the skin on her neck was drooping, causing her to worry that she'd end up with a "turkey neck."

After contemplating plastic surgery for a couple of years, she realized she was ready to take action. She likened her face to "a nice sweater you have that's stretched out and droopy. I thought, gosh, you wouldn't keep wearing that sweater, you'd shrink it up and fix it so it fits better." Amy wasn't interested in making a dramatic change to her look.

"I just wanted to put things back where they used to be with a facial rejuvenation procedure."

Seven weeks after Amy's neck and facelift surgery, she appreciates that her new appearance is very natural looking. "I wanted to avoid that obvious, that I've had work done, because I did this for me. My results look natural, and they feel natural." Today Amy doesn't wear as much makeup as she did before surgery, and she's experienced a big boost in confidence.

All in all, it has surely been a journey of healing with no real issues. However, I am still prone to swelling if I overdo things. Am I happy with the results? On a personal level, absolutely delighted. I still look exactly like me, just less drawn and not so much laxy, crinkly, liney, droopy skin.

I am very pleased, given I am sixty. Scars are negligible, neck droop and jowls gone. I always had reasonably good skin and now it's tighter, not droopy or loose. So yes, I would do it again in a heartbeat. Catch my hubby out the corner of my eye at times and see his quirky smile, he can't believe I actually did it all.

Life is no dress rehearsal and we've each got to make the best of the good, the bad and the ugly—and just keep on trucking.

Elizabeth, a twenty-eight-year-old biomedical engineer, had had quite an unusual reason to consider rhinoplasty (a nose modification).

My heritage is half-Lebanese and half-English. I got a lot of beautiful features from my dad and the Arabic side that I now embrace, like the color of my skin and my eyes.

Many of my features relate back to my heritage, but looking around, nobody in my family had my nose. Growing up, I used to contour my nose like crazy. I never wanted to take side profile pictures and would hate to not be on my good side in photos. I'd look at the photo and focus on how different I looked compared with the rest of my family. I always had this sense of wanting to fit in with my people. I couldn't care less about fitting in with everyone else, but with my family, I wanted to look like I was a part of them.

It took me a while to decide to get this surgery, because when I was younger, my family told me, "No. You were born this way. Nothing will ever be as good as what you're born with." I think a lot of that was ingrained in me, and maybe even the stigma of, "Oh, plastic surgery, you're so plastic." But it's become more socially acceptable. Ultimately it wasn't for anyone else but me.

The plastic surgeon I chose went in and he corrected my deviated septum, and then he also took away that little bump on my nose and the hook that makes my nose point down. Now, when I smile, my nose is straight and actually points up a little bit. He did a really good job in that he didn't make me lose my Arabic or Middle Eastern look.

In conclusion, she relates:

We're about to go on a huge family vacation, and I can't tell you how excited I am to take pictures with them. I sent a picture of myself to my sister just recently, and I was like, "I'm so happy I have your nose now. Now I look like you!" Emotionally and mentally, I was always one of them, and now I look the part.

Lynne, a pharmacy technician, encountered a different concern.

Thinking seriously about cosmetic plastic surgery was initially difficult for me. Over the course of seven years, I had given birth to three wonderful children and spent at least one year breastfeeding each of them. Although I was feeling great about my life, I became self-conscious about my body because of the changes that had occurred from pregnancy and breastfeeding. I began to look at the options that were available to me, and breast implants were the obvious choice.

Lynne then consulted with a cosmetic surgeon, who suggested a breast augmentation procedure.

Choosing to have large implants was a mistake on my part. I should have waited and done more research before making such an important decision. I never felt comfortable with the size of these implants. I did have a discussion about decreasing the size of my implants with the same surgeon after my initial surgery, but this would require an additional surgery that I couldn't afford at the time.

For eight years, Lynne lived with implants she felt were too large.

This time, I went to an actual plastic surgeon who assured me that not only could the implants be removed, but I would be able to regain my breast shape and size with a breast lift.

My surgery was over three months ago, and I couldn't be more thrilled with the outcome. My breasts are soft, beautifully shaped, and much smaller. Prior to my breast enhancement, I would always dress conservatively because I was overly aware of my breast size. I felt self-conscious in certain clothing styles and bathing suits. Now getting dressed in the morning is great; I no longer am constantly trying on various outfits to see what looks okay.

She concludes, "This surgery has made me feel wonderful about my body and myself. I can now go to the gym, swim, and hike without any discomfort. Most importantly, I feel like my body is the correct proportion; I feel and look like myself again."

Samantha faced an opposite challenge. Her breasts were too large.

> The first time I realized I had big boobs was in fifth grade. I'd just switched schools, and my newest friend in class was reminiscing on the first day we met, a month before, when my parents set up a day for me to visit the new school. Apparently, I made a great impression on everyone: I seemed nice, smart, and, according to the boys in the class, was a lot more "developed" than everyone else. I was eleven.
>
> I wouldn't say I *hated* my boobs, but I certainly wouldn't invite them to a party if I had a plus-one. From the day my parents sat me down and told me it was time I get a training bra, I had one wish: smaller breasts.

As Samantha aged, her problem worsened.

> I was 5'1" and officially a 28G, but rarely actually owned a bra with that exact size. Most underwear brands didn't go that far down on the band or that far up on the cup, so I found alternatives—or just opted out of a bra altogether, which was as uncomfortable as it sounds.
>
> Eventually I visited a chiropractor after developing intense lower back pain. He confirmed that I had scoliosis, an abnormal curvature of the spine, and my breast size definitely wasn't helping the pain. I felt validated: My boobs were exactly as much of a burden to my body as I believed them to be.

It was not until her mid-twenties that Samantha made the decision to have a breast reduction procedure. Unfortunately, her postoperative experience was not very pleasant.

> I spent a lot of time in bed the first two weeks after the surgery, with my entire chest wrapped in an industrial-sized Velcro bra.

The pain was bearable, but unlike what I expected: Everything throbbed with a burning sensation that lingered until I was able to take more pain medication.

I couldn't go anywhere that might be crowded, like a bar, or literally any public establishment that posed the risk of someone bumping into my chest. I took Ubers everywhere I could, even though I'd have to lay horizontal in the backseat, cupping the underside of my boobs every time the car hit a bump.

Fortunately, Samantha's outcome proved the procedure worthwhile.

It's now been almost five months since my surgery. I don't have to wear a bra 24/7 anymore, I can sleep on my side again, my nipples aren't swollen, I can run on the treadmill without feeling like a masochist, and boy, do I love being naked. What I see in the mirror is finally what I'd always thought I should be seeing. For so much of my life, I didn't feel like my body was actually mine. Now, I know it is.

Love Yourself First to Love Your Plastic Surgery

Even successful plastic surgery is not going to help you love yourself. Indeed, loving yourself first is a prerequisite for having aesthetic procedures. Clinical psychologists will likely tell you it's possible plastic surgery could worsen your internal anxieties if you are not pleased by your inner beauty. The following are thoughts from women who have suffered from insecurities, negative thoughts, and a perception of body inadequacies. Here are two stories of women who discovered how to love themselves.

Lauren is a writer who discovered a different method to love yourself.

I'm terrible at believing in myself. Whenever a professional challenge or exciting opportunity comes along, my immediate reaction is always "Nope! Can't! Won't!" And yet, when I've completed one of those scary challenges and survived, it's usually the most in love with myself I ever feel. So these days I try to cheer myself on with the kind of unconditional love we give our friends and families, but rarely ourselves.

I know the idea of "dating yourself" has reached the realms of cliché, but I do think there's something in it. When I'm feeling gloomy, rather than slouching about at home, I try to take myself out in a way that feels almost romantic. I plan a lovely day, take myself for a nice lunch, walk the most beautiful route rather than quickest, wear an outfit that makes me feel good, listen to something I love, spend hours cooking an amazing dinner entirely for me.

When I'm feeling like my own worst enemy, I try to treat myself like a best friend I want to spoil, or like a toddler who needs a bit of firm, affectionate parenting. It's about striking that perfect balance, not expecting too much of yourself, but not failing to look after yourself either.

Amika is a nonprofit organizer and has some interesting thoughts on loving yourself.

We're scared to be alone and listen to our own thoughts sometimes. If I'm not talking to my friends, I'm plugged into a podcast, knee-deep in a Netflix binge, or swallowed up by work. Even the simple act of looking out of a window for fifteen minutes allows you to just be and feel.

I can be really hard on myself. I demand too much from my time, and I never think that anything I've done is good enough. My brain exists in a continuous loop of questions about whether I could always have done it better, or in a different way.

Amika sums up her solution.

> Now, I stop thinking about it as soon as it's done, say goodbye to it, let it go for good, and move on. It's taken me some time to learn to do this, but I've stopped picking myself apart in the way I used to.

> Learn to love time alone and apart from other people with nothing but the gentle whir of your thoughts for company. I think putting time to aside to do absolutely *nothing* at all—makes you feel alive and vital.

"Owning our story and loving ourselves through that process
is the bravest thing we'll ever do."
—Brené Brown

Dr. Hardesty: In addition to the good reasons stated to have plastic surgery, none is greater than to help your fellow person and level the playing field. An experience I will not forget was one of my international volunteer trips to Cebu, Philippines. I performed a cleft-lip repair on an otherwise beautiful eighteen-year-old girl. She had been ostracized by her friends and constantly wore a bandana over her face to cover the very obvious facial deformity. When I returned two years later to repair her cleft palate, the girl approached me with a healthy young baby in her arms, tears starting to run down her cheeks. She said, "You made me beautiful. I got married and now have a baby." Yes, a straightforward surgery released her "inner beauty" and allowed this girl to experience a more normal and fuller life.

Dr. Polakof: Self-love is our fuel; it's the foundation for who we are. Everything builds on top of this foundation, and if it isn't solid, life feels shaky. The moment we start loving ourselves, we experience shifts—positive shifts. Life begins to move forward with more ease, and things begin to magically fall into place. Relationships improve. Health improves. And life begins to feel good—really good! If needed to further enhance your inner beauty, this is the time for aesthetic plastic surgery.

PART II

ENTER THE BEAST

CHAPTER 5

BODY SHAMING

"The objectification and scrutiny we put women through is absurd
and disturbing. The way I am portrayed by the media is simply a
reflection of how we see and portray women in general, measured
against some warped standard of beauty."

—Jennifer Aniston

It's difficult to accept, but feeling ashamed of how we look has become normal. Few women believe they have made the beauty grade. We might even think there is something odd about someone who is perfectly happy with how they look.

For some, this anxiety is low-level and periodic—a bad hair day once in a while or a fleeting thought that we wish we could lose a few pounds when we glance in the mirror. For others, it is overwhelming and almost constant, a deep shame which stops us from doing many things important to us.

From famous actresses such as Gal Gadot to pop stars like Kelly Clarkson, there are no limits to the types of people who struggle with body shaming or the way it happens. According to a survey from FitRated, 93 percent of women reported being body-shamed at least once in their life.

Women reported that their bellies and legs were the body parts they most often felt shame about, though they also reported being criticized for their butts and lack of muscle tone or bounce-back after childbirth. The list of where women fail and what they feel ashamed of is almost endless.

Embarrassed about being too fat or too thin. Ashamed of muffin tops, bingo wings, love handles, pancake chests, or flat bums. Humiliated by bumpy, big, fat, and pointy noses. Embarrassed by armpit hair, leg fuzz, and bikini line. Ashamed of cellulite, large pores, wrinkles, freckles, birthmarks, age spots, or pimples.

It's difficult to find a body part which can't be thought of as failing, and flaws—perceived flaws—can be found in every body. No matter how much you might fit the ideal, flaws can be found. Selena Gomez, who was once the most followed person on Instagram, spoke out about how she was body-shamed over fluctuating weight. This certainly contributed to her mental anguish.

As appearance matters more in a visual and virtual culture, our bodies become ourselves, making us completely vulnerable to every form of criticism. This shame is exacerbated and compounded particularly through social media.

Body shaming is ubiquitous; it's part of our routine and everyday experience. We have to be camera-ready—prepared to post our happy families, fun friends, and great colleagues. If we don't get it right, we are fair game, deserving of the snide comment, the snigger, or the trolling. But why? Why does society think it's okay to say negative things about appearance?

It's really difficult to understand why we don't call out comments which make people ashamed of themselves. We call out other negative comments—why don't we call out these? Appearance bullying is the most common kind of bullying and is extremely prevalent.

Effect and solution can be found in the revealing story of **Olivia**, currently a mental health activist, but once a victim of body shaming. She begins by discussing her sad younger years.

> *"Your thighs are too fat." "Your arms are too chubby." "Should you wear that short dress?" "Maybe eat less, you are getting healthy, beta." "Ever tried drinking lemon water in the morning?" "Please go on walks, see how fast you lose your weight."* These sentences may seem like mere statements to you, but to me, they are instances of the times when I was body-shamed not only by strangers or by friends, but even by my own family.
>
> Body shaming starts right from our childhood, with adults policing our diets and outfits—to making comments like *"You are getting really healthy, huh?"* As a child, I have faced body shaming from my friends, teachers. Even my friends have faced the same. My skinny friends have been skinny-shamed and my chubbier friends have been fat-shamed.

Even after Olivia became a full-fledged adult, social image pressure continued.

> I never became aware how real my hate for my body was until I stopped looking at mirrors and started to hate shopping. I hated how my body never looked like that of my friends. I hated how my grandfather thought it would be more appropriate for me to start wearing more "loose" clothes because "fat" people looked good only in loose clothes. These comments scared me so much that even after losing weight I became afraid of wearing fitting clothes.

Olivia began actively dieting, but her frustration continued.

My body issues didn't go away after I lost weight, it only got worse. I started hating and being repulsed of my body more than I should have been. I began counting calories and limiting my meals to such an extent that it made me sick as the days passed on by. I started wearing loose clothes and darker colors just to hide my body.

My body image overshadowed my self-image. I started to starve myself whenever I gained weight, and I rigorously worked out because of this same gain. My stomach was not "flat" enough and for me, my body was never good enough. My body was never enough because it did not look like that of others. I never saw an Instagram model, or a celebrity who had been on magazine covers who looked like me.

Finally, a breakthrough came that changed Olivia's life for the better.

Somewhere amidst the fashion magazines and cabbage soup diets, I forgot to accept my body for what it did. I forgot that my body's job was to keep me alive and breathing. It took me a very long time to accept that my body does everything for me. I learned that bodies are not just for appearance; they are meant for living.

Discovering "**Body Positivity**" taught me to accept my body and to care for it. It made me unlearn the word "fat" and "chubby" as insults. Now I am in a better place. Sometimes, I eat more than I should and regress a bit. But I thankfully have mostly good days and finally am at peace with my body.

> "And I said to my body softly, 'I want to be your friend.' It took a long breath and replied, 'I have been waiting my whole life for this.'"
>
> —Nayyirah Waheed

Learning "Body Positivity" has helped so many women discover their inner beauty and love themselves. The following list can introduce you to healthier, self-satisfying ways of looking at yourself and your body:

Appreciate all that your body can do. Every day your body carries you closer to your dreams. Celebrate all of the amazing things your body does for you—running, dancing, breathing, laughing, and dreaming.

Keep a top-ten list of things you like about yourself. Things that aren't related to how much you weigh or what you look like. Read your list often. Add to it as you become aware of more things to like about yourself.

Remind yourself that "true beauty" is not simply skin deep. When you feel good about yourself and who you are, you carry yourself with a sense of confidence, self-acceptance, and openness that makes you beautiful. **Beauty is a state of mind, not a state of your body.**

Look at yourself as a whole person. When you see yourself in a mirror or in your mind, choose not to focus on specific body parts. See yourself as you want others to see you—as a whole person.

Surround yourself with positive people. It is easier to feel good about yourself and your body when you are around others who are supportive and who recognize the importance of liking yourself just as you naturally are.

Shut down those voices in your head that tell you your body is not "right" or that you are a "bad" person. You can overpower those negative thoughts with positive ones. The next time you start to tear yourself down, build yourself back up with a few quick affirmations that work for you.

Wear clothes that are comfortable and that make you feel good about your body. Work with your body, not against it.

Become a critical viewer of social and media messages. Actually, do pay attention to images, slogans, or attitudes that make you feel bad about yourself or your body. Protest these messages: Write a letter to the advertiser or talk back to the image or message.

Do something nice for yourself. Do something that lets your body know you appreciate it. Take a bubble bath, make time for a nap, or find a peaceful place outside to relax.

Use the time and energy that you might have spent worrying about weight or the shape of your body to do something to help others. Sometimes reaching out to other people can help you feel better about yourself and can make a positive change in our world.

There Is "No Shame" in Calling Upon Plastic Surgery to Assist Inner Beauty

Having a positive outlook about your body does not mean that you cannot choose to make improvements for personal satisfaction. If you believe that having a facelift, breast enhancement, or body contouring will fulfill your desires or gratification, by all means, go for it!

However, we believe it is incumbent upon plastic surgeons to not only foster body positivity, but also make certain their patients are having cosmetic surgery and aesthetic treatments for the right reasons. It is our belief that a focus upon elevating inner beauty should prevail.

Body positivity is a movement that is currently taking the beauty industry by storm and has shifted the landscape of what it means to be beautiful. The movement focuses on building positive body images by promoting the acceptance of all bodies, addressing unrealistic body standards, and helping people build confidence in their own bodies.

While plastic surgery may seem to go in the face of this movement, it doesn't. Instead, it can enhance your inner beauty—and plastic surgery procedures are rising, perhaps because of it.

Our society has for a long time been saturated with images projecting unrealistic expectations of what an individual should look like. Striving toward this hopeless and unattainable standard makes many people experience feelings of self-devaluation or helplessness. As a result, they exhibit unhealthy behaviors and poor mental health when feeling like they are less than enough.

Body positivity promotes the idea that every body type can be celebrated for its unique qualities. This cultivates a healthy and accepting environment that holds no place for body shaming, or plastic surgery shaming for that matter.

Having a positive outlook on your body does not mean that you cannot choose to change it. And if making a small adjustment will cause you to feel more confident and better about yourself and your image, how is that anything but positive?

If you truly believe that facial rejuvenation, a nose job, a tummy tuck, or a Brazilian butt lift will allow you to meet your body goals, then, by all means, go for it! The choices you make for your body are yours and yours alone and should not be dictated by mainstream media, peer pressure, or fear of plastic surgery shaming.

With body positivity, we shift the focus from obsessing over external appearances and obtaining an ideal body to finding a deeper sense of gratification from being healthy and on track. Today, we see celebrities, social media influencers, and online communities coming forward to affirm women's natural beauty.

As a result, many individuals are choosing to commit to the procedures they have long been dreaming of, such as breast augmentation or breast lift surgery. Alternatively, some women who once had breast augmentations are now getting their implants removed or resized for a more proportional appearance. The same holds true for facial and body improvements.

However, we must keep one factor in mind. The reality is that, while plastic surgery is a great way to enhance your appearance and fix poor body image, it can in no way remedy other underlying issues that influence how you feel about your body. That's where the concept of body positivity comes into play.

Ultimately, the motivation to change something about yourself should not be driven by shame or obligation, and it should not be done for the sake of attaining some made-up standard of beauty. Instead, it always should come from the point of realistic hope of wanting to look and feel like your truest self.

Balancing Body Positivity with the Decision to Have a Mommy Makeover

Her name is **Casey**, and she is a mom who believes being beautiful has nothing to do with appearance. She says, "I always believed I was awesome!"

However, life throws challenges at you, and Casey was never one to back down.

> So here I was. Three kids (all C-sections, I might add). My stomach is like a bumpy, saggy, stretch mark-ridden war zone, and my boobs (if I could even call them that) are flappy bags of deflated skin. While I still love myself and am appreciative of all my body has given me, I was over it.

I've worked really hard to lose weight and gain muscle, and I'm ready. I'm thankful for the joy my body has brought, but decided to exchange it for a new and improved one to bring me a different sort of joy. So, I decided to get a "mommy makeover," including a breast lift, breast implants, and a tummy tuck.

While all the planning and daydreaming of my new perky boobs and flat stomach were exciting, I also had to keep in mind I am the mom of two daughters, ages eight and fourteen. I want them to know they are perfect and beautiful and nothing about their appearance should define them.

I think I've done a good job driving home the fact that the content of character and kindness are the true things that make one beautiful. But, at the same time, I hope I have conveyed that I have worked my ass off, and there are some things that I want to improve for myself that I can't do with a healthy lifestyle alone.

So, we've talked about it. I don't get the point of hiding plastic surgery. If anything, I think this perpetuates a culture of morphed body images for younger girls looking to others who have flawless bodies and perfect boobs. I have absolutely no shame in admitting I've had plastic surgery.

Also, since my husband and I basically parent with humor and sarcasm, there are lots of jokes about "Mom's new boobs." That's how I like it. Light-hearted, funny, imperfect. I had plastic surgery to improve my already awesome self. It's all for me, and I think that my girls and family understand that.

Body Image Perceptions Post-COVID-19

The battle in favor of body positivity continues to face challenges. Research published by the *Journal of the International Society for the Study of Individual Differences* reveals that the COVID-19 pandemic actually caused an increase in body image issues.

"Anxiety has risen in adults due to physical isolation and change in routines," according to the study, which claims stressors are also triggering mental health issues such as body dysmorphia and negative body image. Women desire being thinner, and men wish to be more muscular, adding more pressure for people to look a certain way.

The Society's research indicates that some of that negative mindset can come from our phones, especially as screen time increased due to the pandemic. "There appears to be an association between exposure to especially image-based behaviors and content on social media and negative outcomes for body image."

Therefore, it's time to ignore body shaming and get back on track in pursuing body positivity. This is why the Mental Health Foundation says that cutting back time spent on social media can be a huge help if you are trying to become more body-positive.

Limiting your screen time on social media apps can help you adopt new healthier routines. You can use the time you spent scrolling to try new, nutritious recipes or get some fresh air with a short walk.

Let's cast shame on the "shamers" and embrace the fact that inner beauty is the most beautiful component of our lives!

Dr. Hardesty: Unfortunately, shaming and bullying is a real and rampant phenomenon in modern social media. It preys on the normal inadequacies we all felt growing up (and may still have). I personally believe inner and outer beauty combine/morph into one as we understand and appreciate the whole person. True "beauty" is a total package. They not only complement each other, but also enhance our entire being.

I always ask why the patient is having a procedure. If they convey that it's for themselves, then this is a green light to proceed with additional discussions that may lead to a surgical procedure. However, if she says, "Bigger breasts will stop my husband from having affairs," I turn to discussing their misconceptions, explaining that larger breasts won't save a marriage/relationship.

I may well suggest that her funds would be better spent on counseling than surgery. The highest level of intimacy is not physical, but rather a mental state of truly understanding. Loving and giving to each other without any perception of secondary gain is a key element of inner beauty.

Dr. Polakof: The body positivity movement will continue to pave the way for women to feel confident, comfortable, and proud of their bodies. It advocates there is not one standard for beauty, but instead, all bodies are beautiful!

So what does this mean for plastic surgery? Body positivity is an incredible message, one that truly melds well with a woman's desire, independent of outside influences, to improve her body and make the best of herself in her eyes only.

CHAPTER 6

THE IMPACT CELEBRITIES HAVE HAD ON PLASTIC SURGERY AND INNER BEAUTY

"To each his own. I really understand the chagrin that accompanies aging, especially for a woman, but I think people look funny when they freeze their faces."

—Meryl Streep

Have most celebrities benefited from having some type of cosmetic procedure performed? Absolutely! Often, aesthetic procedures have been a boost to their careers. However, we strongly believe that plastic surgery patients must have "realistic expectations."

How Unrealistic Beauty Standards on Social Media Challenge Inner Beauty

Women, in particular, have found themselves battling identity issues due to the unrealistic beauty standards set by what they see on social media. Some have developed serious mental health issues, identity issues, and even body dysmorphia trying to emulate beauty standards that are simply unattainable.

Just as most of us use social media to communicate, tons of celebrities, influencers, models, and brands use it to sell themselves by creating an image of perfection. It's not difficult to see a multitude of perfectly toned beauties, flat stomachs, plump breasts, impossibly long legs, and perky, perfectly rounded butts. Thousands of Instagram accounts promote images of perfectly sculpted women, most of whom are celebrities.

While we may believe we are mindlessly scrolling though such content, our subconscious is soaking it all up, and before we know it, those perfectly formed bodies have become the standard by which we measure everything else.

There is an apparent problem within this false world of perfectionism. Thousands of famous people and models on social media document their workout routines, eating habits, and other aspects of their lifestyle that contribute to the way they look. The problem with this industry is that these depictions are either exaggerated or "fake."

An Instagram model can post a picture of herself in a bikini, showing off her taut stomach, holding up a weight-loss tea supplement. Her caption reveals that said supplement is the secret to her honed physique. This alone sends a very dangerous message to millions of her followers, the majority of whom are impressionable women.

It's spreading the idea that supplements, diet pills, and detox teas are the best way to achieve her body type when, in reality, it could not be further from the truth. More often than not, their looks are a combination of gym, plastic surgery, and a generous amount of photo retouching.

This leads to low self-esteem and negative thinking. It is incredibly important to emphasize to women that social media is not real life. In essence, social media tells us that we need to be a physically beautiful person in order to be worthy, which could not be further from the truth.

There has been somewhat of a beauty revolt, particularly among young, social media-savvy young women. Accounts such as @celebface (revealing the truth behind those "perfect" pictures) have been created to remind us that social media is nothing but smoke and mirrors, and that those we hold in such high self-esteem are nothing but mere mortals.

In order to advance their image and career, many celebrities utilize the skills of a plastic surgeon to assist them in presenting an enviable "picture-perfect" appearance. Some will admit to it and convey they are pleased.

Jane Fonda: At eighty, Jane Fonda is one of the most beautiful women in Hollywood. But the actress is not shy about admitting that she's had help from doctors to achieve her youthful look along the way. The Oscar-winning actress also shared in an HBO documentary that she got plastic surgery around her eyes and jawline because "I got tired of looking tired when I wasn't."

Patricia Heaton: The costar of *Everybody Loves Raymond* isn't afraid to admit she had aesthetic procedures. "I was really in the prime of my career when that was all going on, so it just felt better and made me more confident to reconstruct my stomach, take care of all that stuff." Patricia also shared that motherhood prompted her to get a breast reduction.

Cardi B: Now that she's addressed those perceived issues with plastic surgery, Cardi said she feels "so vindicated." She reveals, "Even when I was eighteen and became a dancer, I had enough money to afford to buy boobs, so every insecurity that I felt about my breasts was gone."

Dolly Parton: She isn't shy when it comes to getting real about the plastic surgery she's undergone over the years. "It is true that I look artificial, but I believe that I'm totally real. My look is really based on a country girl's idea of glam. I wasn't naturally pretty, so I make the most of anything I've got."

Kaley Cuoco: She revealed to *Women's Health* that having a breast augmentation was "the best thing I ever did." The actress, who has also spoken about having rhinoplasty and a round of fillers, also commented: "As much as you want to love your inner self, I'm sorry, you also want to look good. I don't think you should do it for a man or anyone else, but if it makes you feel confident, that's amazing."

However, not all celebrities have good things to say about cosmetic surgery. Indeed, there is something to be learned by flipping to the other side of the coin. Let's meet some forthright celebrities who view aesthetic procedures in a different light than many of their peers.

Nicole Kidman: Academy Award winner Nicole Kidman is an actress known for her timeless looks. "I did try Botox, unfortunately, but I got out of it and now I can finally move my face again."

Tara Reid: Once best known for her role as high school sweetheart Vicky in *American Pie*, Reid is now better known for her bungled liposuction and breast-implant procedure. Her bumpy breast scars, however, weren't as disconcerting as her spoiled belly.

"I had body contouring, but it all went wrong," she said on a broadcast of *The View*. "My stomach became the most ripply, bulgy thing." In a one-word description, the pain she went through as a result of the botched surgery, both mentally and physically, was "horrific."

Jennifer Grey: After her role in the movie *Dirty Dancing*, Jennifer Grey had corrective surgery performed on the shape of her nose. It was a decision the actress came to deeply regret. She called it "the nose job from hell." It changed her profile so much, Grey said that even close friends didn't recognize her. It also took away her "uniqueness," one of the qualities for which she was cast as "Baby" in the film.

"I went in the operating room a celebrity and came out anonymous," she's said since, in acknowledgement of the effect on her career. "It was like being in a witness protection program or being invisible."

Gisele Bündchen: It's difficult for us mere mortals to imagine supermodels like Gisele Bündchen getting insecure about their looks, but it obviously happens to them, too.

The former wife of superstar quarterback Tom Brady, featured on countless magazine covers, Gisele had kids and breastfed them. As a result, she opted to quietly get a breast augmentation, then found she was personally unhappy with her post-augmentation shape. "All I wanted was for [my breasts] to be even and for people to stop commenting on it," Bündchen told *People Magazine*. She said she regretted the surgery almost immediately. "When I woke up, I was like, 'What have I done?' I felt like I was living in a body I didn't recognize."

Gwyneth Paltrow: When you think of Gwyneth Paltrow, you probably think of all-natural remedies to life's issues, including aging, but she has admitted to getting injectable help. "I won't do Botox again, because I looked crazy. I looked like Joan Rivers!"

Courteney Cox: Unlike her *Friends* costar Lisa Kudrow, who has said the nose job she got as a teenager was "life altering," Courteney Cox didn't have such a positive experience getting work done. She says she regrets using injectables to fight aging.

"Everything's going to drop," she said. "I was trying to make it not drop, but that made me look fake... I've had to learn to embrace movement and realize that fillers are not my friend."

Melissa Gilbert: Imagining little Laura Ingalls getting a boob job is probably a shock to *Little House on the Prairie* fans, but that's exactly what happened. She got breast implants after breastfeeding her son left her "enormously insecure" about how her body had changed.

Later Melissa wrote candidly about the experience in a blog post as to how she eventually came to regret them. "Frankly, I'd like to be able to take a Zumba class without the fear that I'll end up with two black eyes," Gilbert wrote, revealing that she was getting the implants removed.

Ashley Tisdale: Singer and former Disney Channel star Ashley Tisdale revealed she had elected to get her breast implants removed. Tisdale said the implants made her feel good for a while, but then the experience turned bad. "Little by little I began struggling with minor health issues that just were not adding up—food sensitivities as well as gut issues...that I thought could be caused by my implants," she posted. "So last winter I decided to undergo implant removal." Ashley also admitted to getting a nose job, which she didn't regret, for health reasons.

Heidi Montag: Reality TV star Heidi Montag became a walking billboard for plastic surgery when she was just twenty-three years old. The memorable figure from MTV's *The Hills* famously underwent ten procedures in a single day. Later, she said it was an ill-advised move, as she almost died during recovery and suffers from long-term health effects as a result.

"I just didn't realize what I was really signing up for," Montag said after she elected to have some of the work reversed. "It just sounds so minor when you have a surgeon describing so much of it to you, like, 'Okay, great, a little of this, a little of that.' You're not told the recovery time and the mental strain that it will put on you, and the long term."

Khloe Kardashian: The entire Kardashian-Jenner family has been pressed on rumors of having cosmetic work done to their bodies, and they've all been pretty open about their experiences. Khloe Kardashian took that honesty to another level when she talked about some facial injections that turned out poorly. On an episode of her show *Kocktails with Khloe*, the media personality revealed, "It did not work for me. I looked crazy... My face was so f—ed, I had to go and get this whole thing dissolved," referring to her fillers.

Reid Ewing: *Modern Family* regular Reid Ewing penned a personal account of his own regrets about plastic surgery. The actor/musician revealed that he battles body dysmorphia, a mental health condition that makes people obsess over perceived flaws in their appearance.

Ewing wrote that he saw four doctors for various procedures, including chin and cheek implants, and not one of them suggested he try therapy. He said that he wished he'd never had any of the work done after realizing the issue was only in his head. "Now I can see that I was fine to begin with and didn't need the surgeries after all."

Yolanda Hadid: A former top model, Yolanda Hadid revealed she's now "Living in a body free of breast implants, fillers, Botox, extensions, and all the other bulls–t I thought I needed to keep up with what society conditioned me to believe a sexy woman should look like. The toxicity of it all almost killed me." Hadid urged her 3.5 million followers to do their research "before putting anything foreign" into their bodies.

Jamie Lee Curtis: Jamie Lee Curtis has been speaking out about the dangers of plastic surgery, as well as social media's obsession with so-called physical perfection. "I tried plastic surgery, and it didn't work. It also got me addicted to Vicodin," the *Halloween* star said in a recent interview with *Fast Company*.

"I was ahead of the curve of the opiate epidemic," she told *People Magazine*. Curtis also said social media can be "very dangerous." She said, "We just don't know the longitudinal effect, mentally, spiritually and physically, on a generation of young people who are in agony because of social media, because of the comparisons to others."

In an interview on *Today with Hoda & Jenna* earlier this year, Jamie opened up about her journey toward confidence and self-acceptance, which is tied to her sobriety from opioids. "My sobriety has been the key to freedom, the freedom to be me, to not be looking in the mirror in the reflection and trying to see somebody else. I look in the mirror. I see myself. I accept myself."

Chrissy Teigen: "I did my boobs when I was about twenty years old," she previously told *Glamour UK*. "It was more for a swimsuit thing. I thought, if I'm going to be posing, laid on my back, I want them to be perky!"

She later told fans, "A lot of people are understandably curious (and nosy!) so I'll just say it here: I'm getting my boobs out! They've been great to me for many years, but I'm just over it."

Then following the procedure, she said, "I'd like to be able to zip a dress in my size, lie on my belly with pure comfort! No biggie! So don't worry about me! All good. I'll still have boobs; they'll just be pure fat. Which is all a tit is in the first place. A dumb, miraculous bag of fat."

There are a number of male celebrities as well who appear to have had poor cosmetic surgery results. This list reportedly includes Sylvester Stallone, Mickey Rourke, Wayne Newton, Ray Liotta, Steven Tyler, and of course, the deceased Michael Jackson.

It's a "Catch-22"

Something that can also often get lost in the frenzy is that celebrities are under more pressure than anyone to conform to impossible standards of beauty. Living under the microscopic lens of the paparazzi and social media, they are taunted and shamed for so-called imperfections and then vilified and shamed when they take steps to live up to the ideal. It's a catch-22 model of beauty, where you're damned if you do and damned if you don't.

No matter what you feel about celebrities, the type of aggressive body shaming that celebrities have been subjected to is toxic—and not just for them. The way we relate and react to celebrities has a huge impact, not only on their psychological well-being but on ours, too. When you start viewing celebrities as a combination of body parts that you are going to be the judge of, the likelihood is that you will end up treating other people in your life and yourself in the same way. With so much of our culture—who succeeds, who is rewarded, who wields influence and power—predicated on appearances, the fascination with the looks of those in the public eye is inevitable. But when you find yourself succumbing to that fascination, the urge to scrutinize every "tweakment" a celebrity may or may not have undergone, and, as a result, how your own face measures up, try to alter the angle of your approach.

Remember that the main purpose of the human body is not aesthetic. Start thinking of your own body—and everyone else's—in terms of all the things it does for you, rather than how it looks. This shift of focus may help you value yourself and others for more than just appearance.

There is a big difference between your aesthetic body and your functional one, but people often forget the functional body they have and focus on the aesthetic. When we focus on the functional—how your body helps you breathe, how it helps you move—that's when we feel much better about ourselves. Something to keep in mind next time you're scrolling through Instagram.

A huge amount of work and money goes into a celebrity's appearance, but because of the lack of information, many may perceive it as natural. But this makes us think, *Why am I so far from this perfect appearance?* However, when you see all the work behind the look, you begin to understand that these celebrities are ordinary people—just like you.

Having relayed these many derogatory reports, it is important to convey that **most celebrities are pleased with their aesthetic procedures**. However, the negative commentaries you have read in this chapter from many luminaries should serve as "warning signs" to consider before deciding upon a cosmetic procedure, and in particular choosing a surgeon.

Dr. Hardesty: Many of the above celebrity commentaries reveal that too often "the enemy of good is perfect!" Celebrities often make their splash when they are young and naturally attractive. However, aging will cause some (with unrealistic expectations) to go to great lengths to recapture what they believe is the look their fans expect.

My philosophy is that plastic surgery can't take you back in time to yesteryear, but rather can rejuvenate your appearance to look as "naturally" good as one should at their age.

Dr. Polakof: While Hollywood and the world of celebrities play a huge role in perpetuating the concept of external beauty, this has little to do with who a person truly is. Beware of the "halo" effect. One great example of the halo effect in action is our impression of celebrity actors. Since people perceive most of them as attractive, it's easy to compare ourselves to physically beautiful actors. However, as you will discover in this book, it is what's inside that truly counts.

CHAPTER 7

A BODY TO DIE FOR?

"Any fool can know. The point is to understand."
—Albert Einstein

Unfortunately, there are a number of doctors practicing cosmetic surgery who have abandoned their Hippocratic oath: "First, do no harm." It is not uncommon for physicians who perform cosmetic procedures to place fortune, fame, and greed before a patient's best interests, turning their medical practices into commercial, marketing machines.

Their "siren song" may be alluring but is often a ballad which can lead to a deadly form of financial seduction and false promises of physical perfection. Is it really worth the quest for physical beauty to risk your life by making unwise decisions about cosmetic surgery and the doctor you choose?

There are some women who have taken such risks to save money and bought into the "pitch" of a notorious doctor without doing their research. Thus, "Buyer beware...it's your life at stake!"

Be forewarned. The following are tragic but factual cases of surgeons and surgeries gone bad. These women did put their lives at risk and paid the price.

Even the rich are not spared from choosing the wrong surgeon. Donda West was the inspiration behind several successful albums and hit singles performed by her son, Kanye West.

Sadly, the fifty-eight-year-old former chairwoman of Chicago State University's English department died the day after her cosmetic procedures. According to the coroner's report, an autopsy found that "multiple postoperative factors could have played a role in the death."

The day after her surgeries, Donda allegedly experienced a sore throat, pain, and tightening in her chest before collapsing in the early evening. A friend at the house called 911, and West was taken to the hospital, where she was pronounced dead in the emergency room.

Certainly, the number of procedures performed during a long period of time under anesthesia might have been a factor. She had a breast lift, a tummy tuck, and liposuction—all during the same time session.

Apparently, other experts with knowledge of West's death point to additional possibilities. One Beverly Hills surgeon told CNN he refused to operate on the fifty-eight-year-old woman due to a heart condition, and this could have been a factor.

Women Seeking Discount Cosmetic Surgery Paid with Their Lives at Clinics Operated by Felons

According to an in-depth *USA Today* investigative news report, body-sculpting procedures have left thirteen dead and dozens injured at high-volume cosmetic clinics.

Nearly a dozen miles from the iconic beaches of South Florida, four convicted felons ran facilities that became assembly lines for patients from across the country seeking the latest body-sculpting procedures at discount prices. And at those clinics, at least thirteen women have died after surgeries. Up to a dozen others were hospitalized with critical injuries, including punctured internal organs.

The owners of these facilities included one man who pleaded guilty to bank fraud. Another was convicted of grand theft in a real estate scam, and two additional crooks admitted to elaborate Medicare schemes that siphoned millions from taxpayers.

The state health department was alerted to the casualties. Government inspectors cited the clinics for serious violations, including dirty operating rooms and sales agents with no medical licenses determining the appropriate surgeries for patients.

At the Seduction by Jardon clinic, hospital records show a thirty-one-year-old woman went into kidney failure and nearly bled to death as she languished in a back room for six hours before her mother found her.

In the New Life Plastic Surgery and Strax Rejuvenation, women died after their doctors injected fat into their muscles in a popular procedure known as the Brazilian butt lift. Medical experts who reviewed autopsies said the fat was injected too deep and collected in their lungs, killing them.

One woman who left Spectrum Aesthetics with a stray surgical sponge sewn into her abdomen later said she would have cancelled her tummy tuck if she knew the operators had been convicted of defrauding Medicare of one million dollars.

A sixty-four-year-old woman was given lethal doses of opioids by her doctor during a facelift, a state malpractice probe found.

Talk about injustice. A manager of the clinic, Evelyn Parrado, was granted permission to run the cosmetic surgery center during the day while spending her nights under house arrest on the felony charge.

The role of these noncredentialed medical clinic operators varies greatly but can include hiring doctors, ordering drugs, scheduling surgeries, and overseeing risk management to cut down on deaths and injuries.

They pay doctors strictly on commission and offer cut-rate prices. As a result, these clinics have packed waiting rooms and busy surgical suites, and at times, gullible, unsuspecting patients must fend for themselves after procedures.

Driven by social media ad blitzes and telemarketers, the clinics continued to grow. They rode the popularity of a new body-sculpting procedure promoted by rap singers and reality show stars like Kim Kardashian: the Brazilian butt lift.

Arizona Cosmetic Surgeon's "Ghastly Shop of Horrors" Investigated After Three Patient Deaths

Dr. Peter Normann advertised quick and easy "lunchtime lipo" procedures at his Phoenix clinic, but the surgeries resulted in three patient deaths.

On a mid-December evening, first responders arrived at Dr. Normann's clinic to find a clinic employee giving thirty-three-year-old patient **Ralph Gonzalez** CPR. Gonzalez had gone into cardiac arrest during a liposuction procedure, and his stomach was severely distended, indicating that the airway tube had been put down Gonzalez's esophagus instead of his trachea. When they arrived at the hospital, Gonzalez's care was transferred to an emergency room doctor, but he was later pronounced dead.

Digging deeper into the patient deaths, it was determined that, before Gonzalez's liposuction began, he was given ten times the lethal dose of lidocaine, causing his oxygen levels to drop and his heart to stop. When the breathing tube was inserted improperly, it only hastened Gonzalez's death.

As the medical board continued its investigation, first responders were called to Dr. Normann's clinic, where they found fifty-three-year-old patient **Leslie Ann Ray** in distress. Her stomach was distended, and she wasn't breathing. Ray was quickly transported to the hospital, where she later died.

Authorities learned that this time, it wasn't Dr. Normann who had performed the liposuction procedure, but a homeopathic physician named Dr. Gary Page, whom Normann had contracted to perform cosmetic surgeries while his practice was restricted.

Since Page wasn't licensed to perform any kind of surgical procedures in Arizona, he carried them out under Normann's direction. It was strictly a cold-hearted monetary reason. After the woman's death, Norman charged her credit card for the full amount of the procedure. Leslie Ray paid for her own death!

CDC Warns Against "Medical Tourism" Plastic Surgery Abroad

Numerous Americans are traveling abroad to save money on medical treatments, a trend dubbed "medical tourism." Many Americans go to other countries for less expensive plastic surgery. However, the Centers for Disease Control and Prevention have issued warnings about seeking medical care in other countries due to potential risks, such as substandard care, exposure to infectious disease and highly drug-resistant bacteria, and an increased risk of blood clots due to flying after surgery.

Recently, a Mississippi woman died after undergoing gastric bypass weight-loss surgery in Tijuana, Mexico. **Markita McIntyre**, thirty-four, died after surgery for a sleeve gastrectomy. She and a friend intended to save money by having this weight reduction procedure done in Mexico. One withdrew from the plan, while Ms. McIntyre, a mother of three, died on the operating table.

Manuel Jose Nunez, twenty-eight, of New York, died after liposuction at Santo Domingo's Caribbean Plastic Surgery Clinic. Manuel Jose Nunez was operated on by gynecologist Oscar Polanco at the Caribbean Plastic Surgery Clinic in Santo Domingo, who has been accused of being responsible for at least three more patient fatalities.

Alicia Williams, forty-five, a teacher from Birmingham, Alabama, also died as a result of complications after a series of cosmetic surgery procedures in the Dominican Republic. After undergoing liposuction, a tummy tuck, and a Brazilian butt lift in the DR, she had several medical problems, including blood clots and loss of a significant amount of blood, before tragically passing away.

A mother of two from California died after undergoing tummy tuck surgery at a clinic in Mexico. **Keuana Weaver** from Long Beach traveled with a friend just over the border to Tijuana for what was supposed to be a routine four-hour operation.

But her mother, Yolanda Weaver, said the thirty-eight-year-old died on the operating table after suffering a heart attack and complications linked to blood clotting. "They discarded my daughter like she was a piece of trash. This just destroyed our family."

Lyndsay Colosimo from Delray Beach, Florida, went to Colombia to get plastic surgery at a fraction of the price that she would've had to pay in the US. Fortunately, she lived, but not without pain and regret.

"I didn't feel good about myself," Lyndsay said. "My dream outcome was to come home feeling better about myself physically. I thought I would be coming home and be able to put on a bathing suit and go run around and look cute."

But her dreams were shattered by complications from the surgery shortly afterward. "I have lost my nipple, and I have an open gash and another wound from where the implant is pulling my skin apart. Dr. Ramos is called the surgeon of Barbies," relates Lyndsay. "I was calling him a butcher by the end."

Even Celebrities Pay a Steep Price for Procedures Gone Bad

The former *Real Housewives of Beverly Hills* star **Yolanda Hadid** has opened up about how her battle with Lyme disease caused her to remove her implants and dissolve her fillers in an attempt to discover the root of her sickness.

"The minute I got on the show, I got sick. I've never worked on that show with a normal brain," she told ABC News. "I was always struggling and always trying to hold on and keep my job."

Yolanda had her implants removed after doctors discovered one implant had ruptured and was leaking silicone into her chest cavity, which she says was aggravating her Lyme disease symptoms.

Crystal Hefner (Hugh Hefner's widow) almost died during cosmetic surgery while having her breast implants removed. "I lost half the blood in my body and ended up in the hospital needing a blood transfusion."

In a story covered by CNN, Crystal Hefner says she "almost didn't make it through" a cosmetic procedure and is using the experience to talk about unrealistic beauty standards. "I should have learned my lesson the first time, but I guess the universe keeps sending you the same lesson until you learn it."

The Sad Story of Heidi Montag

The Hills star Heidi Montag has finally revealed the real reason behind her decision to undergo so much plastic surgery, confessing that her desperation to change her appearance was prompted by cruel comments from internet trolls.

Heidi, who rose to fame at the age of nineteen after appearing on the MTV reality series, which she has now returned to as one of the stars of a reboot, admits now that she regrets the drastic procedures and wishes she had waited until she was older before making such "life-changing" decisions.

"I was just really self-involved at the time—like so many young people— but I was also on TV, where every perceived flaw is amplified. I think I looked in the mirror a little too much," Heidi told *Cosmopolitan Magazine*.

Before being cast in the show. she recalls being "very confident" growing up. However, after becoming a household name, the comments and negativity and hate on the internet began to mount.

It was dealing with that deluge of abuse and criticism every day that pushed Heidi to want to take drastic action to change her appearance once and for all—a move that left her family and friends stunned. Displaying her new look, she announced, "I want to look like Barbie!"

The 5'2" reality star previously recalled hitting rock bottom after she infamously had ten plastic surgeries in one day. Heidi had a chin reduction, brow lift, a second nose job, her ears pinned back, and a second breast augmentation, among other surgeries.

Complications from the surgery almost killed her, and she recalls that she "died for a minute" on the operating table. "My security guards called Spencer [her husband] and told him, 'Heidi's heart stopped. She's not going to make it.'"

"Spencer thought he lost me," Heidi revealed. "With that much surgery, I had to have twenty-four-hour nurse care, and Spencer didn't want to leave my side. I was at a recovery center and had Demerol to deal with the pain because it was so extreme."

Heidi added that "cutting yourself up" is not something she'd recommend. After the life-threatening incident, she found herself at "rock bottom" and had to reevaluate what was important to her.

Reportedly, Heidi is still living with complications from her many surgeries, but her career progresses. There was a reboot of *The Hills* a few years ago, and she continues to appear in movies. Nevertheless, it's a sad story.

Who Will Pay for Your Pain and Suffering?

Nyosha Fowler awoke to a nightmare. A month after an outpatient plastic surgery procedure, the Detroit native's eyes fluttered open. She heard machines beeping and her mother crying out her name. Fowler's abdomen gaped open. And she couldn't walk.

Nyosha learned that her surgeon had accidentally punctured her bowels during liposuction and injected fat into her sciatic nerve during a Brazilian butt lift.

Four blood transfusions and seven surgeries later, the woman was just beginning her recovery when she regained consciousness. By then, her medical treatment costs had already soared over a million dollars.

After insurance paid a share, Nyosha still owed the hospital hundreds of thousands of dollars. She lost her job and was evicted from her apartment. Bills piled up. Her mother connected her to an attorney to sue the doctor.

That attorney, Michael Grife, called Fowler's case heartbreaking—one of the most horrible he'd seen. But there was a hitch: the surgeon was practicing without medical malpractice insurance. Grife withdrew from representing Nyosha because there was little chance she could recoup money for what the doctor had done. She never sued and has been forced to endure years of debt.

Are Doctors Required to Have Malpractice Insurance?

"Going bare" has morphed into an insurance term which means that a medical provider is practicing without professional liability or medical malpractice insurance.

No federal law requires doctors to carry medical malpractice insurance. Whether they are required to have insurance depends upon the state where they practice.

Roughly thirty-two states require no medical malpractice insurance and have no minimum carrying requirements. The other eighteen break down roughly into two groups—states that require minimum levels of insurance and states that require medical professionals to have some insurance to qualify for liability reforms in their state.

For example, nearly 6,900 doctors in Florida lack malpractice insurance or other coverage, colloquially referred to as "going bare," a *USA Today* investigation has found. When they maim and kill, there's less recourse, leaving patients damaged physically and financially, with families struggling to pay medical bills.

While only a handful of states require doctors to carry malpractice insurance, the lack of it creates a serious mismatch with Florida's status as a national destination for discount plastic surgery procedures, including the Brazilian butt lift.

In Florida, one in five board-certified plastic surgeons elect not to carry medical malpractice insurance. That figure does not include doctors who perform plastic surgery without certification, which Florida allows. In turn, this can enable doctors with repeated medical malpractice cases to stay in business without having to pay higher insurance premiums.

By now, you get the picture. Most plastic surgery comes off without a hitch—and most patients tend to be more pleased than not. But aesthetic surgery must be taken seriously, with consequences including death, impairment, and deep debt as a result for those foolish enough to place discounts before safety.

This is why relying on your **inner beauty** is so important. It prevents you from making hasty and less thoughtful decisions about plastic surgery. There is no rush, thus you can take your time to consider options and thoroughly research surgeons. And you don't need to seek out discounts, because you can save up for surgery. Because of your inner beauty, time is on your side.

Dr. Hardesty: Cosmetic surgery won't make you smarter or able to jump higher, but it is designed to improve your self-esteem and confidence. Thus, because it can be well planned in advance, both surgeon and patient can work together as a team to better ensure safe and optimal results.

Most genuine plastic surgeons are capable, experienced, and can be trusted to ensure your safety. The good ones will spend the time to fully discuss possible risks, complications, and options to produce a positive surgical experience and outcome.

Dr. Polakof: Many of the deaths or disfigurations described in this chapter might have been prevented if the patients had more thoroughly examined the surgeon's credentials and experience and researched malpractice suits.

For example, if the surgeon you are considering has ever been sued in your state, there is a record of it. Many of these records are available online, but if they are not, you can pay for a copy. Simply call the clerk's office in the county where the surgeon practices. Additionally, you can contact your state medical board to check for complaints.

CHAPTER 8

WHITE COAT DECEPTION

Truth in Advertising

> "Misinformation is a virus unto itself."
> —Brianna Keilar

It has been referred to as the "White Coat Deception." A number of years ago, the American Society of Plastic Surgeons (ASPS) launched a public information campaign highlighting the dangers of misinformation about "board certification."

In essence, this catchphrase describes the practice of physicians performing plastic and cosmetic surgery without what the ASPS designates as appropriate certification by the actual Plastic Surgery Board. However, in most states, it's legal to perform cosmetic surgery procedures and claim to be "board-certified" in plastic surgery, even though such certification is not sanctioned by the American Board of Plastic Surgery.

While there are no exact statistics as to how many have been misled by such misinformation, we are aware of many tragic misfortunes that have occurred.

The Misfortune of Dinora Rodriguez

Like many women seeking a little surgical assist to remedy a physical problem, this California stay-at-home mom thought nothing of going back under the knife to replace her leaky breast implants.

Sadly, though, Dinora Rodriguez made what experts say is a risky and increasingly common mistake. Based upon her friend's suggestion, she chose a doctor without checking his credentials to ensure he was properly board-certified and adequately trained in plastic surgery. Unfortunately, he wasn't.

The unqualified surgeon so botched the job that Rodriguez made national headlines for the painful deformity he left her with a "uniboob," know in medical terms as symmastia.

The forty-year-old awoke from what she expected to be a simple procedure to find that her new implants were pushed together in the middle, creating one large mass and causing her excruciating pain. If that wasn't bad enough, Dinora also discovered that, without her consent, her audacious doctor had taken it upon himself to "fix" a scar near her eyes, giving her a lift which has since prevented her from closing her eyes.

Experts were in agreement that, because the non-board-certified doctor was not properly trained, he wasn't skilled in correctly performing either procedure, leaving Dinora Rodriguez with lasting medical issues. While her implants can be fixed—though at considerable expense—her eyes cannot.

The scary part is that Rodriguez was far from alone in trusting the wrong doctor. More patients are signing up for plastic surgery procedures performed by physicians with little or no background, training, or certification in the field.

American Society of Plastic Surgeons Expressed Concern

Due to the rampant amount of deception, Dr. Malcolm Z. Roth, a former president of the American Society of Plastic Surgeons, said, "There are dermatologists, internists, pediatricians, you name it, who never held a knife in their training, but in their own office, they are the chief of surgery."

The ASPS was so concerned about this growing trend that it coined a name for this misnomer: the "White Coat Deception" where, in a society that has long revered the medical profession, people believe that just because someone wears a white coat, he or she is up to any surgical task.

But remarkably, despite the dangers, there is no law preventing any doctor with a medical license from practicing a specialty that he or she was not properly trained in. As a result, for many years, the ASPS has been sounding the alarm, which calls for the public to research whether a surgeon performing aesthetic surgery is certified by the American Board of Plastic Surgery. This certification requires a high level of training, superior test scores, adequate experience, and a strict code of ethics.

The Society warns prospective patients not to be fooled by copycat boards with "cosmetic surgery" in the title that do not meet the same standards.

Regrettably, there is nothing to stop doctors who are certified through "weekend courses" from performing procedures like liposuction and offering those services at deep discounts to the public. If prospective patients are not sufficiently aware to research the doctor's background and training, they may be signing themselves up for a nightmare.

A few states have endeavored to clarify the certification issue. For example, several years ago, California ruled that the American Board of Cosmetic Surgery (ABCS) was not equivalent to the American Board of Plastic Surgery.

This cosmetic surgery board is also not recognized by the American Board of Medical Specialties. The standards for ABMS Member board certification and continuing certification reinforce the value of board certification to physicians and medical specialists and patients.

> "We do not see people as they are, but as they appear to us.
> And these appearances are usually misleading."
> —Robert Greene

Today, women in particular are lured by the growing proliferation of advertising promoting a woman's ideal face and body. In addition, some medical practices are marketing a smorgasbord of cosmetic procedures to improve body and facial beauty at cut-rate prices.

Today's consumers are trying to save money, and practitioners are looking for ways to improve revenue. As a result, sometimes at the hands of a less skilled physician, results can be devastating. An attempt to save on the front end can ultimately prove expensive, and perhaps life-threatening, at the back end.

The Real Confusion About Board Certification

In order to better understand the perplexity of certification, let's break down the various medical specialties under which some members perform aesthetic surgery.

Gynecologists are the most utilized practitioners for women. They specialize in women's health, often with a focus on the female reproductive system, and deal with a wide range of issues, including pregnancy and childbirth, menstruation and fertility issues, sexually transmitted infections, hormone disorders, and other female conditions.

Some of these practitioners also perform procedures including breast augmentation, liposuction, and tummy tucks, even though they lack the training and experience of a board-certified plastic surgeon. We have actually heard these physicians ask, "Who knows your body better than your gynecologist?"

They claim to be "board-certified"—and they are—by the American Board of Obstetricians and Gynecologists (ABOG). Thus, these doctors are not plastic surgeons, yet many proclaim in advertising that they perform aesthetic surgery and are "board-certified." True on both counts, except they are not certified by the American Board of Plastic Surgery (ABPS).

Let's turn to dermatology. A dermatologist is defined as "a medical practitioner qualified to diagnose and treat skin disorders." And without question, most derms are very good at skin treatments and enhancements.

Yet a number of dermatologists perform body surgery, such as liposuction. Are they board-certified? Yes, by the American Board of Dermatology—not the ABPS. They do not have the training and experience of a real plastic surgeon.

There is little sense in commenting on the handful of ophthalmologists who perform breast augmentation and body contouring procedures, or a small number of dentists who actually do facelifts. For some unknown reason, their specialty boards do not prevent them from incorporating cosmetic operations in their practices.

Perhaps the most flagrant oddity are those family physicians who perform aesthetic surgery! Believe it, or not, there are some primary care doctors who offer a variety of plastic surgery procedures—both face and body. They too are "certified," in this case by the American Board of Family Medicine—not plastic surgery. But what repercussions might such a clouded certification produce?

Family Doctor Sued by Fifteen Women After Plastic Surgery Complications

Fifteen women sued an Omaha, Nebraska, doctor for botching their cosmetic and plastic surgery procedures, leaving them with excessive scarring, lumps, and pain.

Ironically, *Omaha Magazine* named Gerard J. Stanley Jr. one of the best cosmetic surgeons in the city. But women sued Stanley for causing them pain, suffering, and deformities and misrepresenting himself as a "board-certified" plastic and cosmetic surgeon. The lawsuits claimed that Stanley held himself out to patients as a qualified surgeon, despite not having completed the training for such board certification.

Trish Riddle went to Stanley for a breast augmentation and breast lift, which included liposuction of her stomach fat, which was to be added to her breasts, according to her suit. The surgery, she claimed, left her stomach "saggy and gross," and she said the breast lift didn't work, causing painful lumps and dying tissue in her breasts.

"It's like he didn't even do anything," she said. "It's like I looked better walking in than walking out."

Allison Rockey, an attorney representing another of Stanley's patients, stated that her client received breast implants, a tummy tuck, and a Brazilian butt lift. These procedures left her client with unevenly distributed loose skin and severe capsulation in her breasts, where the breast tissue shrank and tightened around the implant.

"Our expert witness rated the capsulation on a scale of one to four—with four being the worst—as a four. As a result, she was in severe pain. It affected her daily life."

The fifteen women currently suing say they went to Stanley's practice for a variety of procedures, including liposuction, butt lifts, and breast augmentation, only to come away with unsightly and painful damage.

"I mean, they're constantly burning. I have permanent nerve damage in both my arms," one patient stated. Other women allege that their bellybuttons and nipples are misaligned and that they have lumps and scarring.

The website for Stanley's cosmetic surgery center claims that he had received multiple awards for his work. While it's not illegal to perform plastic surgery with only a certification in family medicine, Stanley misled his patients about his expertise and experience.

"They all assumed based on his training, education, and experience that he was qualified to perform these invasive surgical procedures—and obviously he wasn't, because he is only a family practice doctor," said another attorney, James Martin Davis.

After Years of Fraud and Incompetence, an Iowa Surgeon Surrenders His License

After having been the target of hospital sanctions, criminal charges, and fifteen lawsuits brought by Iowa women who claim he left them injured or disfigured, only then did an Iowa doctor voluntarily surrender his medical license.

The case of Dr. Adam B. Smith, then a forty-year-old physician who practiced in Sioux City, illustrates how doctors can remain licensed in

Iowa even as they're accused of fraud, negligence, and incompetence by colleagues, patients, prosecutors, and licensing boards.

"I have to live every day with the pain and mutilation of my body that he caused," one of Smith's patients told the *Iowa Capital Dispatch* newspaper.

Leaving Michigan after a grand jury indictment, Adam Smith traveled to Iowa and was somehow able to join a Sioux City physicians' group named Tri-State Specialists. A few weeks later, Smith was named to the group's Board of Managers, and the Iowa Board of Medicine granted him a medical license.

Within a few months, Smith and a group of other area doctors began soliciting patients for Riverview Plastic Surgery. Court records indicate Smith appeared at a "Ladies' Night Out" event in Sioux City on behalf of Riverview, offering wine, hors d'oeuvres, and "Botox specials" to those who attended. Advertisements for the event stated: *ASK THE DOC! Adam Smith, MD, board-certified plastic surgeon, will be on hand to answer any questions you have.*

In a short period of time, this physician was sued for malpractice by eight Iowa women who claimed they were injured or left disfigured by Dr. Smith.

Concurrently, the indictment from Michigan caught up with him. Soon thereafter, Adam Smith surrendered his medical license, but not before he had left pain and suffering in his wake.

Beware of Label: Board-Certified in "Cosmetic Surgery"

Kathie Pagan's medical troubles began when she underwent an abdominoplasty at the office of Dr. Rouchdi Rifai. An abdominoplasty is more commonly known as a tummy tuck and is performed to tighten the abdominal muscles and remove excess fat and skin. Pagan also received liposuction with the procedure.

The thirty-nine-year-old Jackson, Michigan, woman had been in excellent physical health prior to her surgery, largely because she ran every day for exercise. However, after the surgery, Kathie reported blood clots, dark-colored drainage from the wound, and burning sensations that caused her great discomfort.

With time after the surgery, her ongoing suffering increased, making it difficult for her to even empty a dishwasher. "I wish I would have just treated myself to a vacation and been happy with my body. I would do anything to have my body back the way it was," Kathie said.

After a ten-day trial, the jury found Dr. Rouchdi Rifai liable for breaching his responsibility to meet standards of care. Pagan was awarded $500,000 for disfigurement, scarring, emotional distress, and pain and suffering. The jury awarded her $382,000 for loss of income and $430,000 for loss of future income.

Kathie released a statement stating she is grateful she will be able to provide for her family despite her current inability to work. However, Kathie also noted that no amount of compensation could resolve her lasting medical problems, saying, "I am messed up for the rest of my life for what that doctor did to me."

To this day, Dr. Rifai touts that he is certified by the American Board of "Cosmetic Surgery" and is a member of its sister organization, the American Academy of Cosmetic Surgery. Of course, so are dentists, family medicine doctors, and gynecologists. Thus, do not get this organization confused with the American Board of Plastic Surgery—the certification we recommend.

What Else Can Go Wrong?

Without the expertise of a highly trained, skilled surgeon certified in plastic surgery, a plethora of injuries and deformities are more likely to occur. Here are a few examples.

Because of delicate skin surrounding the eye socket, even the smallest misplaced incision can make a difference. If an eye enhancement incision is made in the wrong location, it could cause the patient to constantly look surprised or cause excess scar tissue to appear.

The use of wrong or outdated breast implants is a repeated reason many medical malpractice claims are brought after breast augmentation surgery. Negligent doctors have been found to use expired, banned, or homemade implants on patients instead of FDA regulated and approved implants. Not only is this dangerous and irresponsible, it is against the doctor's oath to "do no harm."

During an ultrasound-assisted lipoplasty procedure, thermal burns to the skin or other parts of the abdomen caused by the ultrasound probe overheating are possible. Another liposuction complication is necrosis, or dying of cells in the skin tissue, above the liposuction site. This occurs because of lack of blood flow to the area in the event of negligence during surgery.

What Is Unique About a Plastic Surgeon Certified by the American Board of Plastic Surgery?

By choosing a plastic surgeon certified by the ABPS, you can be assured that the practitioner has completed rigorous training and passed comprehensive written and oral examinations covering all plastic surgery procedures.

"Board-certified" means that a doctor's training goes beyond the minimum required for licensure and indicates that he or she has met the requirements of the American Board of Plastic Surgery—the official certifying body for plastic surgeons.

An Overview of the Certification Process

To become a board-certified plastic surgeon, the following is required:

- Board certification by the American Board of Plastic Surgery® (ABPS), or in Canada by the Royal College of Physicians and Surgeons of Canada®

- Complete at least six years of surgical training following medical school with a minimum of three years of plastic surgery residency training

- Pass comprehensive oral and written exams

- Graduate from an accredited medical school

- Complete continuing medical education, including on patient safety, each year

- Perform surgery in accredited, state-licensed or Medicare-certified surgical facilities

- This level of education and training goes well beyond the minimum necessary for earning a license to practice as a doctor, and translates into years of hands-on, real-world training

Note: Most hospitals will only allow plastic surgeons certified by the American Board of Plastic Surgery to perform cosmetic procedures at their facilities.

Why Choose a Board-Certified Plastic Surgeon?

Because training matters. All things being equal, surgeons who train rigorously most often get good results—and an ABPS board-certified plastic surgeon has trained for years before you enter their office as a patient.

Also significant is the ethics course, which is in keeping with ABPS values espousing the importance of ensuring patient safety while providing the highest possible level of care with demonstrated compassion.

Additionally, continuing education is mandatory for a plastic surgeon.

ABPS Continuous Certification Requirements

Part I: Professionalism

- Required in years three and nine of the ten-year certification cycle
- Unrestricted state medical license
- Hospital privileges
- Accreditation of all outpatient surgery centers
- Submission of advertising material
- Peer evaluations

Part II: Lifelong Learning and Self-Assessment

- Required in years six and nine of a ten-year certification cycle
- At least 125 continuing medical education (CME) credits in the previous five years

Part III: Assessment of Knowledge, Judgment, & Skills

- Required in years eight, nine, or ten of the ten-year certification cycle

- Successful completion of the Continuous Certification Examination

- Average pass rate = 95 percent

The Study Guide is available at www.plasticsurgery.org.

Part IV: Improvement in Medical Practice

- Required in years three and six of the ten-year certification cycle

- Completion of one Practice Improvement Module

- Data review of ten patient charts from one operation of your choice

- Review of Benchmarking Report for comparison of data to peers

- Completion of approved educational activity related to selected tracer procedure

- Completion of Action Plan for Improvement

When a doctor is a board-certified plastic surgeon, it ensures that he or she is extensively trained in both facial and body procedures, has learned how to prevent and handle emergencies that may arise during a procedure, and has developed the technical skill and aesthetic judgment to meet a patient's objectives.

Dr. Hardesty: With approximately twenty thousand medical students graduating each year, there are fewer than 180 plastic surgery training positions available. One needs to graduate near the top of the medical school class to even be considered.

Once you are accepted into this highly coveted training position, you will enter residency with the hospital and participate in "on call" duties and graduated supervision for the next six years.

After ten years of medical training (which includes four years of medical school and a minimum of six years of successfully completing postgraduate residency training), the next step in the journey to become a certified plastic surgeon is to undertake a "competitive" qualifying written examination administered by the American Board of Plastic Surgery.

If successful, candidates for certification will submit a list of cases they treated with pre- and postoperative photographs to the ABPS. The board then selects which cases a candidate must present and defend in a rigorous oral test.

Upon being notified of successfully passing the certifying exam, those physicians will join a select group of board-certified plastic surgeons and proceed to benefit from further experience.

Dr. Polakof: Don't be fooled by glitzy cosmetic surgery advertisements and websites or social media prowess. Pay primary attention to whether the surgeon is certified by the American Board of Plastic Surgery.

I strongly advocate that federal legislative action is required to mandate that any doctor claiming board certification must identify the specific board in their marketing efforts, patient literature, and website.

Furthermore, the board they specify must be sanctioned by the American Board of Medical Specialties. For example, this would require a gynecologist who performs liposuction and breast augmentation to specify that he or she is **solely certified** by the American Board of Obstetrics and Gynecology. Let's put an end to certification confusion and bolster patient safety!

CHAPTER 9

HOW SAFE IS THE OPERATING ROOM?

"Little by little, a little becomes a lot."
—Tanzanian Proverb

When performed by a board-certified plastic surgeon, aesthetic surgery is usually very safe. But, as we have seen, misfortunes can occur in the hands of less skilled and greedy doctors.

Here again, when it comes to your safety, attention must be paid to the facility where your surgery will be performed. Careful scrutiny can avoid a variety of little deficiencies which can add up to an unsafe experience.

In today's healthcare environment, surgical procedures may be performed in a variety of settings. Insurance is not generally available for cosmetic surgery procedures, so the high cost of hospital operating facilities means that in-hospital procedures tend to be expensive.

Thus, understanding what to look for in an independent outpatient surgery center is an important consideration for patients, and many factors come into play when examining various options.

Surgical facilities known as ambulatory surgery centers (ASCs) are licensed, freestanding "outpatient" facilities. Such centers are often physician-owned and may specialize only in certain procedures. They are generally well equipped, but typically do not have all the "bells and whistles" that hospitals offer.

Conversely, some contend they are more efficient, provide additional patient comfort, and are, of course, far less expensive than a hospital.

Surgery centers have become increasingly prevalent, and more aesthetic procedures are being performed at such facilities, particularly because of reduced costs. Additionally, advances in anesthesia have improved the safety net for patients.

Conversely, as previously mentioned, board-certified plastic surgeons are generally allowed to perform cosmetic procedures in a hospital, so as a patient, you and your surgeon have the choice. However, as previously discussed, aesthetic surgery is rarely covered by insurance, thus an ambulatory facility will be a far more cost-effective decision.

Having said this, patients who have systemic diseases or medical conditions such as significant hypertension, diabetes, asthma, or other disorders may require inpatient surgery and hospitalization.

Unlike hospitals, surgery centers do not have support departments, such as MRI suites and ICUs, and there have been concerns with regard to their ability to handle major problems, should they occur during surgery.

Since hospitals have more resources to manage complications, patients are often transferred from a surgery center to the nearest hospital facility if serious complications arise during a procedure. Thus, the ease of transfer and transportation should be discussed with your surgeon.

A study on risk factors for major morbidity and mortality from outpatient surgery revealed that patients with cerebrovascular disease, obesity, or cardiac disease or those undergoing prolonged surgery face greater risk, making a hospital generally more appropriate for such cases.

Frail older adults might have stronger reactions to anesthesia and may be more likely to experience surgical complications and take longer to heal; therefore, they should consider surgery in a hospital setting as well.

However, while hospitals are often better suited for higher-risk surgical cases, research has shown that surgery centers actually have certain advantages over hospital facilities.

Due to lower overhead, fixed costs, and the inability of patients to stay overnight, surgery centers often cost 45–60 percent less than a hospital setting. Also, one study revealed that surgery center performance generally exceeds that of a hospital-based facility.

Outpatient surgery centers are able to exercise increased control over procedure scheduling, resulting in reduced procedure delay and rescheduling, and they have been shown to perform procedures more efficiently than a hospital-based facility.

Additionally, although surgical site infection rates are low in both settings, surgery centers experience lower rates on average than hospitals.

Nevertheless, there are downside risks to consider, related to choices.

As Surgery Centers Boom, Some Patients Are Paying with Their Lives

Melinda Van Abbema, a fifty-seven-year-old Colorado teacher, underwent liposuction and a tummy tuck at an outpatient surgery center owned by the surgeon who performed her procedures. But instead of receiving the body she desired, Melinda maintains in a lawsuit that she underwent a nightmare at the center that almost claimed her life.

Melinda contends that the care at the clinic was so deficient that she probably was administered unsafe drugs, causing her to go into acute respiratory and heart failure.

The main culprit apparently responsible for this life-threatening situation was Elizabeth Lammot Campbell, who provided anesthesia services. Campbell had administered anesthetics to Melinda during the surgery, the lawsuit stated.

Shortly after emerging from the surgery, Melinda began coughing up pink, frothy sputum. Campbell then administered Decadron, a drug often used to treat breathing problems.

Melinda reported to the nurses that she felt like she was crawling out of her skin after receiving the medication. She then went into severe respiratory and cardiac failure, according to court records.

Melinda was rushed by ambulance to a local hospital, where she was in intensive care for thirty-nine days. She had to undergo a tracheotomy as surgeons struggled to keep her alive.

The wounds from her liposuction reopened, causing infections and requiring numerous follow-up surgeries. Furthermore, Melinda continued to struggle with ongoing lung complications due to the lack of oxygen she experienced when she went into cardiac and respiratory failure.

In a separate case, the nurse anesthetist, Elizabeth Campbell, admitted to the federal Drug Enforcement Administration that she had stored unsecured drugs in a bag in her car and on a shelf in her garage. The nurse further acknowledged that she may have administered expired drugs to patients, often failing to refrigerate drugs as required, and regularly had drugs handed off to her in parking lots.

Additionally, the surgeon who owned the outpatient center has been sued four times, all of which ended up in settlements, according to state records.

It's Consumer Beware for Cosmetic Surgery in Georgia

The goals were beauty and confidence when patients came, but the results were disfigurement, disability, or death. Dr. Nedra Dodds, who was trained as an ER doctor, performed liposuction and fat injections on a thirty-seven-year-old, April Jenkins, who screamed during the surgery, "It's tearing. It's burning."

A worker stuffed a towel in her mouth so her fiancé in the waiting room couldn't hear the screams. Jenkins ended up dead. A few months later, another patient who came to Dr. Dodds' office for liposuction and fat transfers died, too.

In another Georgia case, Dr. Nathaniel Johnson had his medical license restricted after a patient died during a liposuction procedure. He later lost his license for health care fraud, but that didn't stop him. Police allege the doctor started performing cosmetic surgeries again on unsuspecting patients, using another doctor's name as cover.

In both the Dodds and Johnson cases, these doctors weren't operating in hospitals or licensed surgery centers. They were doing procedures that lasted for hours in their medical offices. In Georgia, that's legal. But that doesn't mean it's safe, according to an investigation by the *Atlanta Journal-Constitution*.

Doctor Who Made Music Videos in Operating Room Hit with Numerous Malpractice Lawsuits

Dr. Windell Davis-Boutte's website called her "Atlanta's most experienced cosmetic surgeon," but a Channel 2 Action News consumer investigation discovered she's had plenty of experience dealing with malpractice cases.

In addition to performing surgery in her office, this dermatologist had posted more than twenty videos on YouTube. Some featured Dr. Davis-Boutte dancing and singing around exposed, unmoving patients.

During one video, she actually made surgical incisions while singing and cavorting on camera.

According to court records, in one of these malpractice cases, Icilma Cornelius came to Dr. Boutte's office for a liposuction and a panniculectomy. It was weeks before the patient's wedding, and she was only a few credits away from earning her PhD. Icilma's mother sadly stated, "She just wanted to be perfect for her wedding dress. My daughter had everything going for her."

Icilma never had the chance to wear her wedding dress or get married. After a more-than-eight-hour procedure, her heart stopped. She suffered permanent brain damage and will require care for the rest of her life.

During her procedure, Icilma Cornelius was not intubated and did not receive general anesthesia. She was given a cocktail of drugs including propofol and fentanyl. The lawsuit claimed no end-tidal CO_2 monitoring equipment was used during the procedure.

Unlike board-certified plastic surgeons, Dr. Boutte did not have hospital admitting privileges, and her Premier Aesthetic Center office in Lilburn, Georgia, was not a licensed surgery center.

Again, this is not illegal in Georgia, and the same holds true for many other states with similar policies.

Be Certain Your Surgeon Addresses Complications and Explains the Steps Taken to Address Them

Here are some of the most common complications which can occur and would be of significant concern, especially in an outpatient facility which is not fully accredited by a national governing board.

1. A **hematoma** is a pocket of blood that resembles a large, painful bruise. It occurs in 1 percent of breast augmentation procedures. It's also the most common complication after a facelift, occurring in an average of 1 percent of patients.

2. **Seroma** is a condition that occurs when serum, or sterile body fluid, pools beneath the surface of the skin, resulting in swelling and sometimes pain. This can occur after any surgery, and it's the most common complication following a tummy tuck, occurring in 15 to 30 percent of patients.

3. **Blood loss** is expected with any surgery. However, uncontrolled blood loss can lead to a drop in blood pressure, with potentially deadly outcomes.

4. **Outpatient surgery infection** remains one of the more common complications of plastic surgery. For instance, infections occur in 1.1 to 2.5 percent of women who undergo breast augmentation. A skin infection called cellulitis may occur after surgery, sometimes requiring intravenous antibiotics.

5. **Nerve** damage potential is present in many different types of surgical procedures. Numbness and tingling are common after plastic surgery and can be signs of nerve damage. Most often, the nerve damage is temporary, but in some cases, it can be permanent. Many women experience a change in sensitivity after breast augmentation surgery, and 15 percent experience permanent changes in nipple sensation.

6. **Deep vein thrombosis** is a condition where blood clots form in deep veins, usually in the leg. When these clots break off and travel to the lungs, it's known as pulmonary embolism. These complications are relatively uncommon, affecting only 0.09 percent of all patients undergoing plastic surgery. Abdominoplasty (tummy tuck) procedures have a slightly higher rate of DVT, affecting just under 1 percent of patients. **Note**: The risk of clots is five times higher for patients having multiple procedures than for those having one procedure.

7. **Organ damage** can occur, particularly at the hands of an unskilled or inexperienced surgeon, during liposuction. Visceral perforations or punctures can occur when the surgical probe comes into contact with internal organs. Repairing these injuries can require additional surgery, but perforations may also be fatal.

8. **Scarring** typically results from some surgeries. Hypertrophic scarring, for instance, is an abnormally red and thick raised scar. Along with smooth, hard keloid scars, it occurs in 1.0 to 3.7 percent of tummy tucks.

Skill and Experience Is Essential in Providing Anesthesia, Particularly in an Ambulatory Surgery Center

Wherever your surgery is performed, you will be given some form of anesthesia or medication to keep you from feeling pain during the procedure. There are four main types of anesthesia used in outpatient surgery.

- **General anesthesia.** This type of anesthesia is given through a mask or IV and causes you to become sedated for the duration of the procedure. General anesthesia is typically used for major aesthetic surgery procedures.

- **Regional anesthesia.** This category of anesthesia is usually given through an injection or a thin tube called a catheter, often in the spine. It numbs a larger part of the body than local anesthetic does, such as your body from the waist down.

- **Monitored anesthesia care or (IV) sedation.** You may be given medication that relaxes you or makes you sleepy through an IV into a vein. Some people are awake and can talk but feel no pain. Others fall into a deep sleep and remember nothing of the procedure. This type of anesthesia is used for minimally invasive procedures.

- **Local anesthetic.** This is usually a one-time injection of medicine that numbs a small area for procedures. You will be awake and alert, but won't feel pain in the area being treated.

It is of significant importance to determine who will administer your anesthesia during surgery. Beware of a surgeon who administers anesthesia while performing the procedure. This can be dangerous, particularly due to the need for constant patient monitoring.

During the actual medical procedure, there are several errors that are frequently made when it comes to anesthesia. These include administering too much anesthesia, which can result in lack of oxygen, brain damage, and possibly death; administering too little anesthesia, which can result in the patient waking up during surgery; administering an incorrect anesthesia drug; and failing to properly monitor all of the patient's vital signs during the procedure.

Additionally, serious complications can occur by using faulty medical equipment and devices that were not tested beforehand—another reason to be certain the ambulatory surgery center is fully accredited.

Who Administers Anesthesia Is Equally Important

Most board-certified plastic surgeons will either utilize the services of a board-certified anesthesiologist or a certified registered nurse anesthetist.

Anesthesiologists are medical doctors, which means they must spend four years in undergraduate studies, four years in medical school, and three to four years in a residency program. Some anesthesiologists may also choose to go on to complete specialty fellowships.

There is a difference to be aware of between a nurse anesthetist and a certified registered nurse anesthetist (CRNA). CRNAs are required to complete an undergraduate degree, become a registered nurse, get one year of critical care experience, then complete a CRNA degree program, which can be from twenty-eight to thirty-six months long. Smaller medical offices are more likely to have nurse anesthetists, while hospitals and larger surgery facilities typically employ both anesthesiologists and CRNAs.

CRNAs have similar responsibilities to anesthesiologists, but in some states they must work with a supervising board-certified physician.

Note: While most patients are fine with their plastic surgeon deciding upon whether to use an anesthesiologist or CRNA to administer their anesthesia, as the patient, you have the right to approve the provider's credentials.

How to Determine if a Surgery Facility Is Safe and Secure

While some minor procedures might take place in a surgeon's office, major cosmetic surgery should be performed in a hospital or fully accredited facility. To be considered an accredited facility, every surgical site where an ASPS member operates must be inspected and approved by one of the following national governing boards:

- American Association for Accreditation of Ambulatory Surgery Facilities (AAAASF)

- Accreditation Association for Ambulatory Health Care (AAAHC)

- Medicare Program, Title XVIII

- The Joint Commission on Accreditation of Health Care Organizations (JCAHO)

The pinnacle of accreditation that hospitals are required to have is by the Joint Commission on Accreditation of Healthcare Organizations, known as "the Joint Commission" or JCAHO. This is a nonprofit organization based in the United States that accredits over twenty thousand healthcare organizations and programs in the country. Furthermore, the commission employs over a thousand surveyors dedicated to improving the quality of patient care.

In addition, surgical centers must adhere to strict principles governing patient safety guidelines, those who operate and provide care in the facility, and sanitation. Accredited facilities must:

- Allow only board-certified or board-eligible surgeons to operate.

- Allow only board-certified or board-eligible anesthesiologist or certified nurse anesthetists (CRNAs) to administer anesthesia.

- Employ only certified surgical technicians, registered nurses, and licensed practical nurses who are trained in the practices of advanced cardiac life support (ACLS).

- Adhere to all local, state, and national sanitation, fire safety, and building code regulations.

- Adhere to federal laws and Occupational Safety and Health Administration (OSHA) regulations, including blood-borne pathogen protection and hazardous waste disposal standards.

- Practice advanced patient monitoring during and immediately after surgery.

Research has shown that accredited ambulatory surgery centers have higher safety standards and better safety records than nonaccredited facilities.

Many accredited surgical centers are also equipped to recuperate patients overnight if the need arises. These facilities have at least two licensed staff members, one with ACLS training, on site at all times, with access to emergency safety equipment and medications. These facilities and staff have clearly defined safety plans which are implemented in the event that a patient requires transfer to a hospital setting.

Dr. Hardesty: The importance of having your surgery performed in an accredited ambulatory surgical center (as above) cannot be overemphasized. In fact, for a board-certified plastic surgeon to become and continue to be a member of the American Society of Plastic Surgeons (ASPS), he/she must agree to and sign an attestation document that they will only operate at hospital/ambulatory surgical centers that have one of the above accreditations.

Again, board-certified plastic surgeons lead in patient safety by committing to the highest level of operating room safety. There are board-certified plastic surgeons who operate in an office-based surgery setting. If this is the case, the designation to verify is the American Association for Accreditation of Ambulatory Surgical Facilities (AAAASF). If the surgeon's facility is not supported by this designation, I strongly recommend that you move on to another board-certified plastic surgeon who can better ensure your safety.

Dr. Polakof: According to *Plastic and Reconstructive Global*: Overall, outpatient surgery has been studied extensively and is safe. The rate of operative mortality associated with anesthesia and surgery in the outpatient setting has been estimated to be 0.25 to 0.50 per 100,000 outpatient procedures.

However, as we have seen, there have been surgical complications due to reckless, inexperienced, or poorly trained practitioners. Tragedies have also occurred in noncertified surgery facilities and due to less qualified anesthesia providers.

A key solution to minimizing surgical risks is to choose a board-certified plastic surgeon who makes safety a priority and appropriately ascertains your risk level. When in doubt, move on to a plastic surgeon you are comfortable with and who emphasizes realistic expectations from his or her patients.

PART III

REVEALING YOUR INNER BEAUTY

CHAPTER 10

SEARCHING FOR DR. RIGHT

"The emotional, sexual, and psychological stereotyping of females
begins when the doctor says: It's a girl."

—Shirley Chisholm

As bombastic as this quotation may sound, there is a great deal of truth in those words. How many male plastic surgeons actually recognize the depth and inner beauty of a woman?

Does this mean women should choose a female plastic surgeon to perform their procedures? The answer is, not necessarily. Rest assured, from our many years of experience, there are indeed a number of male plastic surgeons with the level of sensitivity to discern a woman's inner beauty and perceive her objectives.

Whether the choice be a male or female plastic surgeon, it is the prospective patient who must employ research and intuition to identify a practitioner who best suits their needs, is highly qualified, and falls within an acceptable comfort zone. That will be Dr. Right!

Men comprise 85 percent of board-certified plastic surgeons. Unfortunately, despite impressive qualifications, we are well aware that a number of these male practitioners lack a warm "bedside manner," have an egotistical personality, or may be insensitive to the inner beauty of a woman. For these reasons, we recommend several in-person consultations prior to selecting a surgeon. You deserve warmth, openness, sensitivity, and insight.

Eden is a woman who was interested in a rhinoplasty procedure. Her husband had broken her nose, leaving Eden dissatisfied with her appearance and reminding her constantly of the violence she'd endured.

Eden confessed, "I'd be looking in the mirror at my face and say, 'You look really good today except for your really ugly f-ing nose.' " She continued, "One day I got all ready, did my hair and lipstick, and then I stopped and thought: *Why do you have to feel this way?*"

Eden booked a consultation with a local surgeon who could see her as soon as possible, because she had made her decision and didn't want to wait.

The first doctor she saw—a man—seemed confident he could fix her nose. The trouble arose when Eden began to ask questions. She wanted to know not just *if* he could perform the operation, but *how* he would do it.

The surgeon became annoyed. He got out a mirror and started pointing to the bump and the crooked part of her nose. "I was like, 'That's it? That's the entire consultation?' " she asked.

"It felt like a drive-thru, like you're another female cut-out," she explained. "There was no one asking me what I wanted to look like, what I wanted to accomplish. I remember he said, 'Don't worry. We'll make your nose real sexy.' And I thought, *I'm not coming to you to be sexy.*"

Should you consult with a plastic surgeon as Eden has described, don't walk out—run! Regardless of the quality of the credentials, this type of egotism and insensitivity is simply unacceptable.

In any case, the first prerequisite in finding a plastic surgeon to consult with is to perform research—and do it **thoroughly**.

Advertising Can Be "Way" Misleading

Cosmetic surgeons have increasingly come under fire for using advertisements that may be deceptive or intended to solicit vulnerable consumers.

The marketing and advertising of cosmetic surgery in the United States has become a controversial issue. This arises with the normalization of unrealistic beauty images in the media and of consumer self-diagnosis. In addition, more and more surgeons are using aggressive marketing tactics to promote aesthetic procedures and prey on the insecurities of prospective patients.

Social media has become a home base for false claims. For example, according to an *Aesthetic Surgery Journal* study, only 18 percent of practitioners advertising aesthetic surgery services on Instagram are board-certified plastic surgeons.

The Journal research team reports, "The scarcity of actual board-certified plastic surgeons amongst the most-viewed cosmetic surgery posts on Instagram is alarming."

Even Big Media Can Be Fooled

Kay, a second-grade teacher in Chicago, beat cancer at the age of fifty-six and decided to do something nice for herself. She kept hearing about a Beverly Hills plastic surgeon. He was on *Good Morning America* and Fox television, and was featured in *People* magazine. She called his office and asked if he could "tuck" her upper eyelids—then boarded a flight to Beverly Hills.

According to Kay, that was the beginning of a two-year nightmare. She recounts that the surgeon and his staff manipulated and misled her from the start. He talked her into doing both upper and lower lids.

Kay reports that when she awoke the morning after surgery, there was no feeling in her left leg. The next day, her bandages were removed. She was shocked to see that he had cut around both ears—which were still being monitored for cancer—and her chin.

Kay had merely wanted to touch up her eyelids, but instead had been subjected to major cutting. Dazed, she considered her options. "I'm two thousand miles from home, I'm all by myself, and I've been slashed."

When Kay returned home, she decided to more thoroughly investigate the surgeon and was surprised to discover that there had been twenty-four previous lawsuits brought against him. This included a wrongful death suit and one brought by a woman who claimed the doctor had left a scissor piece in her body.

Kay continues to wake up several times a night with excruciating pain and has hearing loss, facial scarring, and nerve damage in her leg—not to speak of psychological scars. Of course, the major media that touted this surgeon's sterling reputation never covered Kay's story—nor those others.

The Never-Ending Deceptive Marketing Tools

Cosmetic surgery is a big moneymaker, especially for those greedy, unethical, pretend-to-care physicians. From "doctored" before and after photos on social media to professionally written patient testimonials, it's difficult to know what to believe. There are even awards and endorsements that cosmetic surgeons can purchase, as well as posting made-up testimonials.

Understanding the Aesthetic Procedure That Best Reveals Your Inner Beauty

As important as choosing Dr. Right is, understanding the aesthetic procedure or procedures which can meet your facial or body improvement objectives—and that showcase your inner beauty—is equally important.

1. Identify your specific objective, or objectives, and write them down to preserve your focus during your search for Dr. Right.

2. Perform an objective self-evaluation. Where in your face, or on your body, do you see a need for improvement—and **why?** Remember, you should be seeking these improvements for yourself—not others.

3. Are you both physically and mentally healthy—and are your expectations for improvements realistic? What if the outcome of surgery falls short of your objectives? Can you accept only a slight enhancement?

4. Begin researching those procedures which can best meet your objectives. The more you are educated in aesthetic procedures of interest, the better prepared you are to choose a surgeon.

5. With its many advertisements and self-serving links, the internet can be confusing and not a good place to start. Fortunately, Part IV of this book will provide you with excellent information regarding the key aesthetic procedures—along with insightful input from patients.

You may also wish to visit the website of the American Society of Plastic Surgeons: www.plasticsurgery.org. The primary purpose of the ASPS site is patient education. Their "Cosmetic" section clearly identifies each area of the face and body as well as surgical and minimally invasive procedures. Under "Find a Surgeon," you can also locate board-certified plastic surgeons in your area.

Again, don't make a big mistake by thinking it's as simple as turning on your computer, typing in "plastic surgeon near me," and calling the first doctor you find who seems like a decent fit to perform the procedure you've been longing for.

Choosing Dr. Right should involve a good deal of research, knowledge, and ultimately consultations. After all, the surgeon you select will alter your appearance for the rest of your life.

Number One Priority: ABPS Board Certification

As we conveyed in Chapter 9 ("White Coat Deception"), certification by the American Board of Plastic Surgery is essential to making certain your surgeon has the necessary education, training, and experience to perform cosmetic procedures capably and safely.

To ensure further safety, based upon their ASPS membership, these plastic surgeons must operate in fully approved facilities, as also described in Chapter 9.

Beginning your research based upon these important criteria will quickly eliminate doctors who are less qualified and are not required to adhere to such safety standards.

What to Look for in Patient Reviews

While it is a good idea to go to a surgeon's website to get a feel for his or her practice, the vast majority of sites will, by and large, only publish information the marketing arms of these practices want you to know.

Patient reviews fall into this category. It is unlikely that a surgeon's site will post unfavorable reviews; thus we recommend two relatively independent resources.

Healthgrades—An Independent Source of Information

According to a study by *USA Today*, Healthgrades is the leading comprehensive physician rating and comparison database for every major medical specialty. Along with comprehensive data about a doctor's qualifications, it's important to know what real patients say about their experiences with a provider. We find that Healthgrades takes a series of steps to protect the quality and integrity of patient reviews. All reviews are confirmed and audited before publication. Community members have the ability to flag inappropriate content for further review by their team.

We should also note that doctors cannot pay for good reviews, nor can they pay to have negative reviews removed. Additionally, any reviews that are deemed fraudulent or violate their guidelines will be removed immediately.

Dr. Polakof: For purposes of physician privacy, we chose to use Dr. Hardesty's Healthgrades profile to exemplify what this review resource provides.

Dr. Robert Hardesty, MD Cosmetic, Plastic & Reconstructive Surgery •Male •
Age 68 • 54 Ratings

Imagine Plastic Surgery 4646 Brockton Ave Ste 302, Riverside, CA 92506

Dr. Robert Hardesty, MD, is a cosmetic, plastic, and reconstructive surgery
specialist in Riverside, CA, and has over forty-three years of experience in the
medical field. He graduated from Loma Linda University School of Medicine
in 1978. He is affiliated with medical facilities such as Loma Linda University
Medical Center and Redlands Community Hospital.

About Me: As a board-certified plastic surgeon, my greatest concern is for the
safety of my patients. I work only with certified anesthetists or anesthesiologists
who are with you monitoring your vitals and assuring pain-free surgery. I work
only in accredited surgical centers and hospitals.

Dr. Hardesty's Reviews

Likelihood to recommend Dr. Hardesty 4.4

Based on 54 ratings—45 Five-Star Reviews

Sample Patient Review: "Dr. Hardesty and staff are amazing!! They make you
feel comfortable and welcome, and they address your fears and concerns like
you are their only patient. They make you feel like a person and not patient
xyz. Dr. Hardesty even said a little prayer with me before my procedure which
brought me a lot of comfort because I was nervous the day of my surgery. I had
no complications after getting my implants as I was worried about capsular
contraction, but Dr. Hardesty went over how he does the operation and how he
uses the Keller funnel to reduce the risk of that occurring. I highly recommend
Dr. Hardesty. I'm so pleased with my natural-looking breasts and with the care
I received. I really felt like part of the family."

However, Dr. Hardesty also had negative reviews. Here are condensed patient
criticisms: "Staff wasn't friendly" (6) "Difficult to schedule appointment" (2)
"Office environment average" (2) "Long wait times" (2).

This site continues by providing Dr. Hardesty's background, the hospitals he is associated with, and their patient ratings, along with other helpful information.

Healthgrades also offers quite a bit of additional information—for example, a background check: "No malpractice claims found for California." The site also rates the hospitals where Dr. Hardesty has operating privileges.

RealSelf: Complete Focus on Cosmetic Plastic Surgery

RealSelf primarily targets plastic surgery and dermatology, with more than thirty thousand registered doctors and practices. It's a forum where consumers can share their experiences, and the site has more than two million reviews. (Reviews can only be removed if they violate the terms of service.)

Note: RealSelf verifies that reviewers are true patients; thus they are allowed to post anonymously under a pseudonym. However, for a monthly fee, the company will boost content about a surgeon which has no relationship to the validity of reviews. The site also offers substantial educational information about aesthetic procedures.

Social Media and Other Types of Reviews

With Facebook and Google, there is no verification process; thus, anyone can leave a review. In general, social media reviews simply cannot be trusted.

Review companies may be somewhat helpful, but they are businesses that often charge doctors for greater visibility. The documentary *Billion Dollar Bully* shows the darker side of how Yelp operates.

So why not ask your primary care doctor or specialist for an opinion? It's a good idea, but keep in mind that, while doctors may have heard good things about a plastic surgeon, often they will not be familiar with his or her actual results or patient satisfaction.

Again, the very best option for authentic reviews is to speak with a surgeon's patients (which will be covered in the following chapter). However, visiting the reviews site that we recommend is a good start.

Are Top Doctor Awards Valid?

In short, the majority of Top Doctor awards are paid programs, meaning that physicians can pay for the distinction of being listed even if they have little legitimate medical merit to back it up.

Reporters from ABC uncovered a particularly unsettling story. In a shocking instance of medical malpractice, a neurosurgeon allowed an instrument to slip and damage the brain of an elderly woman during surgery. She died several weeks later. Despite this incident—and with over a dozen medical malpractice suits against him—the doctor remained listed as a "Top Surgeon" by the Consumers' Research Council of America.

Having said this, awards generated by peer votes have more credibility. Essentially, these organizations will poll a large sampling of physicians in an area and ask them what doctors they would recommend for certain specialties. Doctors can usually only choose one physician and can't vote for themselves. After the results come in, the organization will analyze which doctors were recommended the most by their peers and present them as top doctors.

For example, **Castle Connolly Top Doctors** designations, which cover all fifty US states, are based on nominations from doctors themselves. They ask physicians to consider many criteria when nominating their fellow providers. The premise is simple—as a doctor, who would you go to if you needed care?

Their physician-led research team then thoroughly screens each nomination to ensure that every Top Doctor selection meets Castle Connolly's rigorous standards. Top Doctors do not pay to receive this designation.

Another legitimate quality-of-care resource is the "Best Doctors" designation for a plastic surgeon. Their large number of voting physicians helps eliminate the conflicts and biases of smaller-scale surveys. Additionally, Best Doctors never accepts compensation or gratuities of any kind from physicians.

An interesting honor designation is the "Compassionate Doctor Award" by Vitals, another large physician review resource. This award recognizes doctors who treat patients—not just conditions—with care and grace. In a recent Vitals Index survey, one out of three respondents said that a doctor who "listens and spends time" with them was the most important quality indicator.

Compassionate Doctor Award winners are chosen based on the number of reviews a doctor receives from patients for the calendar year and minimum rating values. The algorithm also takes into account other quality metrics that the provider must meet.

Lastly, if you wish to be fully diligent in your search, query the state medical board about the surgeon (or surgeons) of interest. State medical boards are the agencies that license medical doctors, investigate complaints, and discipline physicians who violate the Medical Practice Act. A list of state boards' contact information is offered by the Federation of State Medical Boards, www.fsmb.org.

Be mindful of the fact that a malpractice suit does not necessarily mean the doctor has been negligent or done something illegal. However, if you are impressed with a surgeon, be certain to request his or her response regarding any malpractice suits during your consultation.

Surgeon Websites and Photo Galleries

Most plastic surgeon websites tend to be attractive—and if not, perhaps you should question the surgeon's aesthetic taste. However, while endeavoring to be informative, the vast majority of these sites are primarily designed to market a surgeon's services.

The surgeon's photo gallery, where before and after results photos for various procedures can be studied, should be of particular interest to a prospective patient.

Of course, it's entirely possible that results can be Photoshopped to appear impressive—and you would need to have an expert eye to detect manipulation. The good news is that, if a surgeon is a member of the American Society of Plastic Surgeons (ASPS), Photoshopping or retouching a patient result would be a violation of their code of ethics, which can result in severe disciplinary action.

Here are some tips on viewing before and after pictures.

Examine Before Images Which Most Resemble Your Age and Needs

Look for consistency—not "cookie cutter" results. The most highly skilled plastic surgeons will adjust their technique and the surgical outcome to complement each patient's unique anatomy and match their personal preferences. A sign of such skill is a gallery where results look different, but almost all of them look attractive and natural with that patient's features.

On the other hand, if a surgeon you are considering has some very nice results, but all the patients appear much the same in the after photos, it suggests that this particular surgeon is very good at achieving one certain look. Unless that appearance matches what you want, it may be best to consider a different surgeon.

Symmetry Should Be Maintained and Improved

Most people have some natural variations in symmetry. Sometimes this is slight, but other times it is severe. While a plastic surgeon may not be able to achieve perfect symmetry with a procedure, a skilled practitioner will work to improve symmetry between features and balance among features.

Scars Should Be Placed Strategically

An experienced plastic surgeon will place incisions in the natural folds of the skin or where they can be easily concealed by clothing whenever possible.

Look at Before and After Photos Both on the Surgeon's Website and Again During Your Consultation

Most plastic surgeons keep digital or print photo albums of their patients' results in their office which contain many more photos than they place on their website.

This will also enable a surgeon to explain their approach to achieving a good postoperative result. Additionally, the quantity of pre- and post-op pictures can indicate his or her level of experience with that procedure.

Contacting Practices and Your Decision to Schedule a Consultation

Once you have narrowed down plastic surgeons of interest, the final step in your research process is to contact those practices for further information. Avoid inquiring through email, because you will rarely receive more than generic responses that do not provide insight into the practice.

When calling, request to speak with the patient care coordinator or patient counselor. Briefly describe your procedure (or procedures) of interest and ask the following questions:

- Verify that the surgeon is certified by the American Board of Plastic Surgery.

- What is the general estimated cost of the procedure(s)?

- Does the cost include the operating facility, anesthesia, and supplies?

- Where does the surgeon perform his or her surgery?

- What specific accreditation does the surgery facility have?

- Does the surgeon utilize a board-certified anesthesiologist or a certified nurse anesthetist (CRNA) to perform anesthesia?

- Based upon your procedure(s) of interest, what is the expected recuperation period (downtime)?

- How many of these procedures has the surgeon performed? Also, how many during the past year?

- Have the coordinator describe the surgeon's level of sensitivity with his or her patients. What is his or her "bedside manner" like? These questions may initially stump some coordinators, but this will often enable you to ease into whether the surgeon is capable of recognizing your inner beauty.

- Evaluate the patient coordinator's knowledge, demeanor, and willingness to be helpful—thoroughly answering all your questions without being defensive. The coordinator is a reflection of the surgeon and his or her practice—particularly since this person has been appointed the primary source of contact with new patients. It's not a "deal-breaker"—but worthy of consideration.

There are other items you may ask about, such as financing, postoperative care, openings for surgery, and more, but these are important questions which will assist you in determining whether you wish to consult with a particular surgeon.

In conclusion, plan to consult with at least three board-certified plastic surgeons prior to making a final decision to have surgery.

Dr. Hardesty: In my opinion, choosing surgeons to consult with in finding "Dr. Right" should require time, effort, and patience. You need to carefully evaluate credentials, experience, and reviews, as well as before and after pictures on surgeon websites.

And definitely book at least three consultations. Each consult will provide the surgeon's perspective as to your needs and realistic expectations in respect to results. Likewise, you will experience the "cultural" component of the office. Is it an assembly-line operation and "one size fits all"?

Or do the surgeon and staff take their time to discuss options and present all phases of the aesthetic journey—particularly, identifying your needs from an "inner beauty" perspective?

Lastly, there are the financial considerations. Here, you must keep in mind that this is your body, and you are worth it!

Dr. Polakof: Should you decide to proceed in booking a consultation with a surgeon, there is often a consult fee. Don't be reluctant to ask—since you are serious about having the procedure(s)—whether the coordinator will agree to waive that charge. Don't allow a consultation fee to prevent you from meeting with a good surgeon, but there is no harm in asking.

Finally, with many practices, virtual consultations are available. You may wish to take advantage of this option, particularly if you are prepared to travel for your aesthetic surgery. However, if at all possible, it is advisable to meet with a surgeon personally, in his or her practice environment, prior to making a final decision.

At least be certain to perform thorough research and speak to a few of the surgeon's patients in advance of surgery.

CHAPTER 11

MEETING DR. RIGHT

"Everything has beauty, but not everyone sees it."
—Confucius

Now that you have diligently performed your research, it's time to pick and choose. This means preferably consulting with at least three board-certified plastic surgeons. Will one—or all—recognize your "inner beauty"?

Be mindful that—since these are likely well-qualified surgeons—after all your questions are answered, you want to be certain that your "inner beauty" has been recognized and that surgical recommendations are based upon these unique qualities you possess. In any case, here is generally what to expect.

On the days of your consultations, dress comfortably and avoid heavy makeup. After all, if inner beauty is to be discovered, you want to be "you." Also, don't forget to bring a complete list of prepared questions with you.

Typically, you will first meet with the patient coordinator, who will introduce the surgeon and ultimately quote surgical costs, as well as make arrangements should you later decide to choose this practice for your procedure. "Later" is the operative word, since you should always take time to carefully consider all factors prior to your final decision.

Usually, a plastic surgeon will first examine you before initiating the consultation. This will also be your first opportunity to examine his or her level of sensitivity and "bedside manner." Normally, he or she will attempt to make you comfortable by asking questions about you.

The physical examination phase may also be a good time to express your interests and objectives, clearly explaining that having a cosmetic procedure is not based upon how you might appear to others, but instead, for personal satisfaction, how you feel inside.

Take the time to tell the surgeon a bit about yourself. If the doctor is truly interested in your feelings, they will delve deeper with questions of their own. This may be your first clue as to whether a good fit is possible.

Your Consultation with the Surgeon

The next step will entail the surgeon explaining his recommendations for the aesthetic procedure (or procedures) which will serve your objectives.

Be wary if the surgeon endeavors to promote additional procedures which are unexpected. It's possible there are good reasons for suggesting additional options, but there are some surgeons who do this primarily for financial gain.

Oftentimes, the surgeon may promptly address procedure complications, as well as benefits. At this point, he or she may also offer before and after patient photo examples to review with you.

In any event, after the review of patient photos is the time for your prepared questions. While most prospective patients are a bit nervous at this stage, put yourself in the position of an employer interviewing a potential employee applicant. You may be surprised by how much this positioning empowers your confidence.

If, for some reason, the surgeon has not shown you before and after patient pictures, begin by requesting them. Reviewing pre- and postoperative photos will enable you to study the surgeon's expertise as he or she explains their approach and technique involved in creating those results.

Additionally, the number of pre- and postoperative examples shown may also be indicative of the surgeon's experience with a procedure.

New considerations may arise, but here is the prepared list of questions to inquire about (in your own preferred order).

Note: Some of the questions you likely asked when initially speaking with the patient coordinator, but it's important to hear the surgeon's perspective.

- How many times have you performed this surgery during the past year?

- Based upon what I wish to accomplish, why will the procedure(s) you recommend help me achieve my goals?

- How safe is the surgery? What are the possible complications?

- Where will my surgery be conducted? What safety precautions are in place at that facility?

- Do you have hospital privileges to perform my procedure should I prefer this option? If so, which hospitals?

- If for some reason a serious complication occurs during surgery, which hospital would I be taken to—and how far is it?

- Have any of your patients had serious negative outcomes? Also, have you been involved in any malpractice suits?

- What are the certifications of the person who will administer my anesthesia? How long will I be under general anesthesia—or anesthetized?

- What about scarring? Will scars be visible? Can they be minimized?

- Are there nonsurgical options for what you are recommending?

- How long will my recovery last, and what will it be like?

- What kind of pain should I expect, and how will my pain be managed? Is there someone I can call if there are problems?

- What activities can I do during recovery? When can I return to work?

- How long will the results last? Will I need future "touch-up" treatments?

- If revision surgery is necessary, will there be an additional charge?

- How many revisions have you found necessary for this procedure?

- Do you carry supplemental insurance for your patients in case of problems? (Some practices offer programs such as CosmetAssure.)

- What are my options if I'm dissatisfied?

At this point, you need to once again review your objectives with the surgeon. Then ask: "Are you confident my objectives can be met—and do you feel my expectations are realistic?"

As the surgeon answers each question during your consultation, it's important to be an intent observer. Remember—you are the employer. Closely evaluate his or her strengths and weaknesses. If he or she becomes defensive in response to questions you pose diplomatically—consider moving on. Likely, your relationship will only worsen.

Hopefully, the surgeon will be respectful—impressed by your preparation and sincerity. And, hopefully, he or she will recognize your inner beauty shining through.

Your Interaction with the Patient Coordinator

The vast majority of plastic surgeons choose not to discuss costs or surgical arrangements, and after the consultation will suggest you meet privately with the patient coordinator.

Keep in mind that, although the coordinator (almost always a woman) is trained to be helpful, her most important task is to book surgery. Thus, patient coordinators tend to be sales-oriented in a "subtle" manner.

After briefly discussing your procedure(s) with the surgeon, she will often prepare a written quote for surgery and review costs with you. Carefully study the expense breakdown and verify that, in addition to the surgeon's fee, facility, anesthesia, laboratory, medications, and all supplies are included. Specifically ask if there are any other costs, including charges before and after surgery.

The coordinator will probably have already mentioned that financing can be arranged through an outside company (e.g., CareCredit). But due to the competitiveness of the plastic surgery field, there is often a bit of room for negotiation. It's always best to negotiate from a position of strength.

Advise the patient coordinator that you have many family members, friends, and business associates who will be anxious to see your results, since some may be interested in an aesthetic procedure of their own. Then ask if discounts are available. Oftentimes, in the eyes of this staff member, you are now a potential referral resource and perhaps worthy of a discount.

Note: More big savings might be available if the surgeon has a cancellation. An opening in the doctor's schedule, as well as the operating facility, motivates the practice to promptly seek a patient replacement. This usually presents an opportunity for a significant discount. Should you later decide to choose this surgeon, ask to be placed on their cancellation schedule.

When the patient coordinator asks if you have any questions, this is a good time to make your request to **speak with practice patients** who have had a procedure similar to what you are considering. Even if the procedure(s) the surgeon recommends is unique, still ask to confer with surgical patients.

Body Language Is a "Telling Tale"

Body language not only indicates how surgeons feel—consciously or not—about a patient, it impacts your perception of the doctor as well. Known for his pioneering work on nonverbal communication, Professor Albert Mehrabian of UCLA reveals that interpretation of a message is 7 percent verbal, 38 percent vocal, and 55 percent visual. The conclusion was that 93 percent of communication is nonverbal in nature.

Most experts agree that at least 70 percent of all communication is nonverbal, underlying the importance of noticing body language. Thus, your observation of a surgeon's nonverbal reactions during the consultation likely demonstrates his or her interest in your personal perceptions and objectives.

There are some surgeons who are so confident in their opinion as to what is best for a patient that your feelings are of lesser importance. There are signs to consider. During the consult, did the surgeon consistently make eye contact with you or often look away? Did he or she appear somewhat impatient (tapping a pen, talking at a fast pace, often changing positions, sometimes with arms folded in a stance of protection) as opposed to being open and welcoming?

From harsher voice tones to forced smiles, there are body language signals that the surgeon believes he or she knows best and is somewhat perturbed by your large array of questions. These types of communications through body language should be a red flag in your column of "Cons."

T-Square Your Pros and Cons

Following consultation appointments, you will want to list the strengths and weakness of each plastic surgeon, including your feelings about support staff. Ultimately, there will come a time to compare surgeons and their practices.

In order to simplify and better organize these tasks, we suggest utilizing the T-square approach. On either a sheet of paper or a file on your desktop PC, laptop, or notebook, create a line across the top with a line or space down the middle. Below the surgeon's name, enter *Pros* on the left side and *Cons* on the right.

Following each consultation, and while impressions are fresh on your mind, list all the positive aspects about the surgeon under "Pros" and negative perceptions under "Cons." Also include your feelings about the practice and staff.

Questions to Ask Yourself

Obviously, your hope is that each surgeon will patiently and openly respond to your questions, providing knowledgeable, helpful, and reassuring information.

When examining before/after procedure photos and listening to the explanation as to how he/she created the result, did you gain an impression of creative artistry or simply basic competence? Are the surgeon's aesthetic improvements subtle, or do they proclaim that patients had cosmetic surgery?

Did he/she provide a good explanation of your procedure(s) and confirm that surgery would be performed safely in a secure environment with the likelihood of few, if any, complications? Is the recovery time acceptable with your work or lifestyle schedule? In respect to your satisfaction with results, did he/she provide an acceptable answer? Did staff members seem supportive?

And, as importantly, did the surgeon make an emotional connection with you? This means, did he or she listen empathetically and communicate an understanding of your individual needs and desires? Was your inner beauty warmly and supportively recognized?

The final step is to speak with a few patients of the practice to inquire about their impressions and satisfaction. Those patients provided by the coordinator will obviously be pleased with results, thus your inquiries should be focused on their deeper insights.

Assuming they are quite satisfied with an improved appearance, ask questions such as, "What were your objectives prior to having surgery? Did you experience much pain, and how was your recovery period? What did you find "unique" about Dr. X? What was the worst part of your experience during and after surgery? If you could suggest any way Dr. X or his staff could improve patient experiences, what would that be?"

As you review your T-square surgeon comparisons and move toward a final decision, affordability is generally the last important consideration. It's a challenge for many but reminds us of a quote from singer-songwriter Jill Scott:

> You owe it to yourself to
> live beautifully. And I am.

During their lifetimes, most good people sacrifice much for others. Every so often, it's time to do something nice for ourselves. If the price of having a quality physical enhancement to complement your inner beauty is a bit steep, there are options.

Most practices can lead you to reputable surgery financing companies which offer low, affordable monthly payments. Most of these programs do not have prepayment penalties, meaning you can pay the debt off at any time to reduce interest fees.

The most important aspect of deliberation is not to make your final decision in choosing a surgeon based upon cost. There is much truth in favor of the old adage "You get what you pay for." This is your body—and you owe it to yourself not to compromise on quality.

Fortune may come your way, and the surgeon you choose may offer the most favorable cost—or you place yourself on their surgery cancellation list and later realize substantial savings. In any event, you are doing this to please yourself and deserve the very best!

Does Plastic Surgery Make People Happy?

Research published in *Clinical Psychological Science* reports that plastic surgery patients often experience more joy in life, a higher sense of satisfaction, and greater self-esteem.

The study's authors looked at first-time patients and compared them to people who had always wanted plastic surgery but ultimately decided not to go through with the procedure.

When comparing psychological test results of the surgical patients with those who had not had plastic surgery, people who had cosmetic procedures experienced higher self-esteem, had less anxiety, and felt healthier overall. Additionally, those who opted for a procedure reported they were happier with their bodies as a whole, not just the area on which they had work done.

Stories of Lady J and Lady Q

We wish to share the stories of two women who had facelifts and are very pleased (actually "thrilled") with their results. For purposes of privacy, we shall call them Lady J and Lady Q. Both are intelligent, successful women.

Lady J, at the age of fifty-six, decided to investigate having a facelift for two very explicit reasons.

> Primarily, I wanted a facelift for my career, and secondarily, I wanted to look on the outside the way I felt on the inside.

> As a woman in an industry dominated by men, I began to feel like I was beginning to be passed over for them—or for younger female colleagues. Professionally, I was really just hitting my stride and was very good at my work.

> Like it or not, it was clear to me that I needed to look younger if I was going to continue to compete at the highest level of my profession. Secondly, I'm an active lady, a workaholic and physically fit. I sure didn't feel the way I looked.

Lady Q had a similar yet different reason for pursuing a facelift.

> I had my facelift at the age of fifty because my looks did not reflect who I was. Forever a fitness fan, my body still looks great, but my face has always been droopy, sad, and tired looking.

Looking in the mirror, I always thought I was sad or in a bad mood. My eyelids were like window shades and always looked old. It is just how my family looks; we have droopy, loose skin. I actually had my facelift done ten years ago, but I continue to be so happy with how the surgeon made my face reflect on the outside who I am on the inside. I am beyond thrilled how it turned out in such a beautiful and natural way!

"Improving upon my looks became a research project," said Lady J.

I began investigating nonsurgical treatments at a well-regarded dermatology office. Wanting to learn about fillers, lasers, and other nonsurgical, cosmetic stuff, my visit to the dermatology office left me very dismayed. Frankly, the staff at this office drank way too much of their own Kool-Aid! I didn't want to look like any of the women in those offices. I did not want a Hollywood face. I wanted a younger, well-rested, and completely natural look.

Lady J's search led her to a board-certified plastic surgeon's office when she learned about a surgery done for a woman who had had an excellent result following a traumatic facial injury. "She looked phenomenal," said Lady J.

In turn, Lady Q described what she liked about the aesthetic specialist. "I know for a fact my surgeon strives to be a perfectionist who will not cut any corners to hurry the time spent with any patient, either in the office or in surgery."

Mary—A Mommy with a Makeover

Mary recounts what motivated her to turn to cosmetic surgery.

After my pregnancy, I just felt unsure about myself. I was a newly single mom with this wonderful little girl, but my self-esteem was just gone. I didn't feel like myself, and I was completely self-conscious.

I did my research and consulted with a plastic surgeon who made me feel completely comfortable. We were even able to joke together. Ultimately, we decided upon a mommy makeover.

Now I'm more confident than I've ever been, and I know that people can see that I now feel like my inside—who I really am—matches my outside.

My biggest motivation was my daughter. I knew she looked up to me, and I wanted her to see a confident person. She was picking up that I didn't feel good about myself even when I was smiling and pretending that I was. I am now so proud of myself, happy, and excited—I even have more energy. Because I feel good about myself, I know it benefits her too.

Yes, the surgery was a big expense for me, but it was completely worth it. If I had to do it over again, I'd do it in a minute—I actually wish I had had it done three years earlier, soon after my pregnancy—I feel that good about the results.

In conclusion, you'll be surprised how many patients had cosmetic surgery procedures to have their physical appearance better match their inner beauty. When doing this for the right reasons and carefully choosing your plastic surgeon, you will likely feel good about yourself, as well.

Dr. Hardesty: Nothing can replace a face-to-face meeting with your surgeon, but I am a fan of an initial telemedicine consult. Why?

- Patient convenience (time and efficiency), plus a preliminary interaction with your prospective surgeon.

- Objective review of patient self-generated photos in a protected HIPAA electronic environment.

- Both the patient and the plastic surgeon "get a feel" for each other and see if they are a good fit to work together.

If you click, absolutely schedule a follow-up with an "in-person" appointment.

FYI: What I like to tell my patients is this: "I earn my living by operating. I earn my reputation by not."

Dr. Polakof: Several years ago, a New York city plastic surgeon wrote the following:

> The word "beauty" is the most overused, misunderstood, poorly defined word in the English language. What makes a woman beautiful? The Holy Grail of beauty has never been completely understood. The cliché "Beauty is in the eye of the beholder" is incorrect in my opinion. Perception is the key. It is "perception of beauty" that is in the eye of the beholder. Each of us, however, has a different perception of beauty.

Good point. During your consultation, why not ask the plastic surgeon about his or her definition of "beauty"? This may be an indication of whether you at least somewhat see eye to eye. It's worthy of a discussion.

PART IV

PLASTIC SURGERY ADVANCES AND PATIENTS

Meet Patients Who Honestly Discuss
Their Procedures

CHAPTER 12

FACIAL REJUVENATION

"No matter how many faces I have,
there is no changing the fact I am me."

—Kobo Abe

Facelifts: Achieving the "Natural Look"

Note to Readers: Commencing with this chapter, the reader will begin to see QR codes, which will reveal Dr. Hardesty's actual patient before/after photographs. The link can be accessed from smart phones with a QR code reader app or by taking a picture of the code.

 Most people think about getting a facelift in their late forties or early fifties. Around that age, facial features undergo a significant change due to volume loss, as well as loss of fat in the cheeks. This results in deeper "smile lines" that run from the nose to the mouth.

Also, this is often a drooping effect that continues down to the jowls, which changes the appearance of the face.

The traditional or surgical facelift is also called a rhytidectomy. This is performed to reposition the soft tissues of the mid and lower face and neck into a more youthful and refreshed contour. Facelifts address several problems areas, including sagging cheeks and the deep creases between the cheeks and the lips, drooping jowls that muddy a crisp jawline, and excess skin and fat on the neck.

The greatest compliment any plastic surgeon can receive are the words, "I can't believe it: the results look so natural." But the hard truth is that not all plastic surgeons achieve the natural-looking results that patients desire—especially when it comes to facelifts.

A common misconception is that plastic surgery is noticeable. The truth is that great plastic surgery is invisible. When it is performed properly, patients should look natural and beautiful or handsome, yet totally untouched.

Specific facelift procedures will address and treat many concerns on the face such as "turkey" neck, neck bands, jowls, and wrinkles from excess sagging skin, excess skin, dense grooves from the base of the nose to outer lips, and sagging cheeks. The specific facelift technique is used with other adjunctive procedures, such as fat grafting, laser, and orbital rejuvenation, providing what we refer to as "synergy."

The goal in using these combined procedures in a comprehensive plan is to have you look ten to fifteen years younger in a natural way. Depending on the type of facelift needed, your surgeon should utilize hidden incisions that, when healed, will be virtually unnoticeable.

Using these small access sites around the ears and under the chin will tighten the underlying muscles, elevate the skin, and remove the excess skin and tissue that causes premature aging, sagging, and dense lines.

Then the muscles and underlying tissues are tightened, and the skin is gently redraped without tension, resulting in a natural sleek and youthful appearance.

By having a properly designed facelift, you are rejuvenating your facial features and returning to a more youthful and natural appearance.

Your surgeon should take precautions to position the incisions in the most inconspicuous locations. Here are various facial rejuvenation options.

Mini Facelift

Small incisions may be made at key locations along the hairline and ear. This is best for early signs of facial aging.

Mid Facelift

A tiny incision in the temporal scalp hair and a small intra-oral incision is all that is usually needed. This is an approach often utilized for isolated droopy cheeks.

SMAS Facelift

Depending upon the treatment area, the incision may be located along the hairline behind the ear or along the ear/face junction and extending under the sideburn area. A small hidden incision is often made under the chin. This is the most common type and versatile facelift procedure, addressing all components of the aging face, such as droopy cheeks, jowls, and sagging neck.

Subperiosteal or Deep Plane Facelift

This procedure often combines the incisions of mid facelift and SMAS facelift. It's best for elevating and repositioning sagging muscle groups.

Meet Two Facelift Patients

Theresa had a full facelift procedure, including eyes, twenty years ago.

> I had never even considered plastic surgery until I caught a glimpse of myself in the mirror and saw my mother. She was very pretty and always looked younger than her years, but she had her eyelids done, and it really boosted her self-confidence.
>
> That is when I realized I had the same droopy eyelids she had. I was fifty at the time and thought it wouldn't hurt to explore the possibility.

Once Theresa studied her face carefully, she noticed that simply addressing her eyelids would not be sufficient, and she decided to have a facelift and browlift along with surgery for her upper and lower eyelids.

She speaks frankly about her surgery and postoperative period.

> I think I was as prepared as possible. The pain was probably more than expected because it is hard to imagine pain. But the medications made it as comfortable as can be expected. There was a bit of an issue in one lower eyelid, but it was addressed immediately and healed nicely.
>
> This being twenty years later I still do love the outcome. I should mention that I had a touch-up "tuck" on the facelift just last year, and I continue to be very pleased.

After seeing Theresa's results, her husband, Steve, also chose to have a neck lift. "I wanted to get rid of my hereditary turkey gobbler. All my relatives on my dad's side have it, and I didn't want to keep it. My confidence level is much greater, and I am often told I look younger than my age."

Bob's Mini Facelift

In addition to Theresa's husband Steve, there is another gentleman with proof that men also recognize their "inner beauty" needs. **Bob** states, "There is nothing more subjective in life than the reflection we see when looking into a mirror. Regardless of what friends, family, or life partner may tell us, what we see in the reflection is how we define our appearance."

Bob, who had a mini facelift, continues, "Hopefully our appearance is not viewed in the extreme as how we define ourselves as worthwhile individuals, but certainly self-esteem and confidence in everyday life helps us to simply feel good about ourselves."

Bob has some advice for men and women who postpone their interest in self-improvement. "Most patients always say that they should have had the procedure done years ago and why did they wait so long? Sooner rather than later in life—treat yourself to your choice of enhancing cosmetic surgery."

The Case for a Neck Lift

Many like Steve and Bob find that excess skin tissue on their neck mars their appearance and causes them to look much older than they are. The "turkey wattle" is an uncomplimentary feature that many wish to eliminate.

The neck lift helps to tighten the muscles on the neck while removing excess skin and fat. This method is more isolated than that of a general facelift, and it helps to contour the jawline for a younger appearance.

The neck lift is often done in combination with other procedures such as a facelift, cheek lift, or facial liposuction. All of these procedures help to visibly change signs of facial aging. The incisions used in the neck lift procedure will be made in inconspicuous places so that, when healed, they are virtually unnoticeable.

Benefits of a Forehead Lift

The forehead lift, also called a brow lift or browplasty, is a procedure that helps to rejuvenate the brow area and forehead to attain a younger appearance. Every year, thousands of people undergo this procedure and receive natural yet amazing results. Forehead lifts are designed to reduce sagging skin and prevent wrinkles and fine lines that appear on the forehead, between the eyes, and on the bridge of the nose.

As we age, our skin begins to lose collagen, which helps to maintain the elasticity of our skin. In turn, this results in the brows sagging. The more the brows sag, the more your forehead muscles try to raise them, and thus the wrinkles appear.

This is an unfortunate circle, resulting in drooping brows (due to continued loss of collagen and elastic fibers) which result in additional forehead wrinkles. The increased collagen and elastic loss causes the brows to drop, resulting in further wrinkles from overworked forehead muscles—and the circle continues.

At times, when looking into the mirror, you may feel you appear tired, sad, or grumpy simply because your brows are sagging. By having your brows lifted, you break the circle of wrinkle formation. With brows in a normal position, a youthful and alert appearance is most often regained.

Additionally, your forehead muscles aren't constantly contracting, thus fewer wrinkles or lines will appear across your forehead.

Eyelid Enhancement

"Beauty is how you feel and it reflects in your eyes."
—Sophia Loren

 Our eyes are perhaps the most important features of our face. It's one of the ways we telegraph our moods, emotions, and feelings. Unfortunately, over time, our eyes may begin to look tired, sad, and droopy. Even when we are well rested, that bright, "wide-eyed," youthful appearance is missing.

Eyelid surgery, known as blepharoplasty, can enhance appearance and self-confidence, rejuvenating the "windows of your soul" with a bright, refreshed outlook and presence.

Eyelid surgery can be performed on either the upper lids, lower lids, or both. After a thorough examination of your bone structure, facial muscles, and the symmetry of the eyebrows, your plastic surgeon will formulate a customized treatment plan for you.

Upper Eyelids: The incision line will be placed at the natural eyelid crease. Then the excess skin, bulging fat, and muscle will be removed. A post-op ultrasound might be used to help with swelling and bruising.

Lower Eyelids: Typically, the incision is made just below the eyelashes. The trimming of fat and excess skin will take place as well as tightening of the lower eyelid muscle. An alternative option, when there is minimal excess lower eyelid skin, is to place the access incision on the inside of the eyelid.

Beatrice was motivated to have a blepharoplasty procedure due to droopy eyelids inherited from her mother. "I always had a 'surprised' look due to raising my eyebrows to lift the eyelids. As I aged, these 'defects' seemed to become more pronounced."

Her top priority was to first find a well-trained, skilled plastic surgeon who was highly experienced in eyelid surgery. She did a good deal of research. "I required my surgeon to be personable and pleasant. To treat each question as though it was meaningful and not stupid. To look inside me and see the real me...not just another face to improve." Beatrice found him.

"The actual surgery went beautifully, but I had a complication no one could have foreseen. I did not know that I was allergic to the epinephrine in the lidocaine. My face blew up like a balloon. I was transferred to an ICU for the night until my swelling subsided."

Beatrice is pleased by the final outcome. "Shortly after having the cosmetic surgery, I attended my high school reunion—no squinting or frowning! No 'surprised' look on my face! I feel amazingly satisfied with the long-term results. People continually remark on what a youthful face I have and the inner glow that just shines through."

She has good advice for those considering cosmetic surgery. "Be realistic in your expectations. But most of all, do it for yourself...because that's who counts in the long run!"

Eyelid Surgery and Insurance

The vast majority of cosmetic surgery procedures are considered "elective" and not covered by insurance. However, if upper eyelid skin is blocking your vision, surgery may be judged non-cosmetic and perhaps entitled to insurance coverage. The rule of thumb is that, if your eyelid surgery is done for functionality improvement, then it may be considered reconstructive and insurance-worthy.

After a consultation with your selected surgeon, discuss this possibility with the patient coordinator. She may be able to help facilitate a request to your insurance provider to see what the company will cover.

A Nose Like Any Other Nose

Before getting into the art of rhinoplasty, we would like to share **Jackie's** story, since it provides interesting perspectives.

"I never really had a problem with my nose when I was younger," claims Jackie. "I was always told I'd taken after my Greek dad, with my slightly bulbous tip and a crooked bridge, but it gave me character."

She continues, "But in my late teens, I found myself caught up in the social media storm. Suddenly, I was spending hours on end scrolling through Instagram, being bombarded with snaps of beauty bloggers, makeup artists, and models with picture-perfect features—and mine didn't match up."

Jackie finally decided to take the plunge.

> I don't really remember the pain or the black eyes, but I do remember crying myself into a state over how my nose looked after the cast had been removed. I felt an overwhelming sense of disappointment.

> The plastic shield had pinched my tip. The swelling made me look like something out of *Avatar,* and I was terrified that I'd be haunted by the regret of my expensive decision. What had I done to my face? Did I look better before?

Relief soon came.

But as time went on, the swelling began to subside, and my nose finally started to look like it belonged on my face. A quick catch-up with my surgeon also revealed that it takes longer for those with "thick skin" (a certain characteristic of Mediterranean and Middle Eastern noses) to see the swelling subside. It can even take up to a year, sometimes longer, for your nose to assume its final shape.

Jackie makes the point that it doesn't matter what other people think.

Nose jobs aren't meant to completely change your face, and a reputable surgeon will tell you that good plastic surgery should make it impossible to tell whether you've undergone a procedure at all. To me, my new nose finally looked like it belonged on my face. I was in love with it.

She also makes the point that rhinoplasty won't change the way people perceive you. "My straighter nose gave me a new lease on life—a newfound confidence—and I was certain it'd land a boyfriend, too. But I've realized that if a guy is going to ghost you, he'll do so regardless of your looks or sparkling self-assurance."

We find that Jackie's concluding words provide good advice to prospective patients.

Long story short, if you waltz into the surgeon's waiting room and tell him you want a "Kim Kardashian nose," chances are, you won't walk out with one. An honest surgeon will explain that you can't ask for someone else's nose. It simply won't suit your face."

The Beauty of a Nose— Rhinoplasty

 Nose surgery, medically referred to as rhinoplasty, can help to improve both the functionality and appearance of your nose, if you have issues with breathing due to a deviated septum (the partition between the left and right nose openings) or overly large turbinates, which can decrease the ability to breathe through your nose.

A septoplasty (straightening the deviated and crooked septum) and turbinate reduction could benefit you immensely.

If you have a crooked, large, unshapely nose or a bulbous tip, an experienced plastic surgeon can help you obtain the nose you desire. Should you also need functional as well as cosmetic improvements of your nose, both concerns can often be performed at the same time under one anesthesia and recovery period.

Procedure Options:

- **Silicone implants:** If there is not enough nasal cartilage to use for the augmentation of the nose, a silicone implant may be a viable option, though it comes with more side effects since it is a foreign object being used.

- **Autologous cartilage**: These are grafts taken from the nasal cartilage. If unavailable, ear or rib cartilage can be used as well. This option offers the best chance for long-lasting, natural results, since it's your own tissue.

- **Fillers**: Some fat grafts or fillers may be used as well to smooth out any lumps on the nose.

Incision Options

Open rhinoplasty: These incisions are typically made along the tissue strip that separates the nostrils. This technique provides a direct approach to the underlying boney and cartilaginous support tissue, and the incision is almost imperceptible when healed.

Endonasal rhinoplasty: These incisions are usually made completely inside the nostrils. Thus, there are no external incisions, and all supporting tissue is not directly visible.

With respect to recovery from a rhinoplasty procedure, usually within a week, bruising and swelling subsides to show the refined appearance of the nose. At this time, splints are removed and the results from nasal surgery are apparent. During this time period, you can usually return to normal daily activities.

For the first six weeks after surgery, non-contact, non-high-impact, and limited but progressive exercise can occur. Often, over time, the nasal shape subtly continues to improve. It may take up to a year to see the full results from a rhinoplasty procedure.

A Case of Resolved Insecurity

Kaylee was insecure about her nose as long as she could remember, with negative whispers beginning at a young age.

> Whether the comments were about my nose being big or looking "witch-like," these remarks from grade school stuck with me into adulthood. I remember times in college when I had to make video presentations, all I would be able to focus on was how my nose looked throughout the video.

As the years progressed, her perception worsened.

> As camera phones and social media gained popularity, I would then consistently see photos of myself and fixate on what my nose looked like. This fixation would ruin the moments captured and take me from being present because my mind would be stuck on my nose.

> There were several things I did not like about my nose. It was large, had a bump, and would droop down when I smiled. It also never seemed proportionate to my other features and overall face.

Finally, she had had enough and began visiting plastic surgeons whom she hoped could fix her problem.

> What I was looking for was someone who took the time to talk to me and showed care for me as a whole person, not just a potential rhinoplasty patient. But some surgeons tried to talk me into more procedures. They felt more like sales people instead of caring about me and my concerns.

> I chose a surgeon who made me feel comfortable and heard. I never felt rushed with that doctor. I had tons of questions, and he took his time in answering all of them. He would write down answers, provide visuals, and made sure I was thoroughly educated in the process with realistic expectations.

Kaylee had a positive surgical experience because she was well informed as what to expect. "I had a cast for about a week and needed to tape my nose for some time. I liked that my surgeon and his staff were very supportive. They called often to check on me, and I had multiple office visits in which I was carefully examined."

Today, Kaylee is pleased she has a proportionate nose in harmony with other features—and has advice for others with similar interests. "Educate yourself and know your options. Get multiple opinions and as much information as you can. Make sure you are making decisions for yourself and not for others."

She encourages introspection. "Learning to be happy with yourself, confident, and doing inner work is all an equally important part of the process. Do what makes you the best possible you."

Beautifying Your Features with Facial Implants

There are many who feel that their features aren't proportionate or wish to enhance their definition. They opt to have facial implants placed in such areas as the cheek and chin.

Facial implants are designed to reconstruct and rejuvenate your facial features. The implants are available in a wide range of sizes and styles to help restore contour and proportion to the face. The facial implants can help with your lips, chin, jaw, and cheeks. Many patients desire a more projecting jawline or to permanently plump up their lips. Some wish to enhance fullness in their cheeks and/or to help correct any facial asymmetry.

Reshaping Your Ears

Some people have been self-conscious about their larger ears for years. It's a shame, because many celebrated individuals—such as Hollywood hunk Channing Tatum or Will Smith, who claims he has the perfect ears to play former President Obama in a movie—are not bothered by their noticeably big auricles.

Both Jennifer Garner and Jennifer Aniston have been pinpointed as having larger-than-normal ears. It's a personal choice, but if you are bothered by having bigger ears, there is an aesthetic solution called otoplasty. This surgery helps reduce large ears, shape ear lobes, correct disproportionate ears, restore prominent ears to a normal position, and restore after ear loss. It's also helpful for those who have had injuries to their ears.

Otoplasty creates a more natural shape and look. Thus, if the size of your ears is bothering you, or your child is having issues, a skilled plastic surgeon can create a more desired aesthetic look. (Children above the age of five are able to undergo this procedure, since this is when the ear cartilage is stable enough for correction.)

With both adults and children, an incision is made behind the ear that is hidden and when healed is almost imperceptible. The cartilage in adult ears is harder, so it is mechanically softened. This enables the permanent sutures to hold and allows for repositioning.

Recovery from surgery usually means remaining at rest for a few days after the procedure. After this time period, you can return to normal daily activities without any dressings or bandages.

Brian and Prince Charles

Brian had an otoplasty procedure some twenty years ago.

> My ears stuck out prominently, not as bad as Prince Charles, but enough that it bothered me since elementary school. I was never teased, but I just didn't like the way my ears stood out.
>
> It was one of the best decisions—of any kind—I have ever made. I'm very happy with how they look. Nobody in my family really noticed. None of my friends noticed. It was a seamless transition.

Dr. Hardesty: My goal has always been to perform surgery which is largely undetectable to the outside world. In my opinion, surgeons should be more concerned about preserving a patient's privacy and creating an improved "natural" appearance, which primarily provides personal satisfaction.

Creating a natural outcome in facial rejuvenation is based on understanding each patient's unique anatomy and then bringing forth inner beauty, which results in an enhancement that is mainly inconspicuous.

Dr. Polakof: One of the biggest fears about having cosmetic surgery is to not look like yourself after a procedure. We have all seen that obvious plastic surgery appearance with a person's face looking too tight or pinched.

From aging Hollywood actresses to strangers at the supermarket, there are a large number of women who seemingly choose surgeons who go too far in their attempt to reverse sagging cheeks and jowls or recapture youth.

The main goal of facial plastic surgery is not to dramatically change how someone looks, but rather to enhance and rejuvenate a person's appearance.

CHAPTER 13

NONSURGICAL FACIAL REJUVENATION

"By looking at only one place, you miss everything in all the other places! Look everywhere to see everything!"
—Mehmet Murat ildan

You should absolutely look for less invasive options to achieve your facial and body goals. Sometimes surgery is necessary for a good result, but many times, there is a viable option to consider.

According to American Society of Plastic Surgery statistics, over the past decade, there has been a dramatic increase in the demand for noninvasive rejuvenation procedures. Part of the upsurge in noninvasive procedures can be attributed to the rise in new injectables and technologies now available to plastic surgeons.

Many of the soft tissue fillers, laser treatments, and radiofrequency and ultrasound-based skin tightening methodologies used today were introduced within the last decade. With the growing availability of novel techniques, plastic surgeons are charged with maintaining a masterful knowledge of how to deliver these interventions to optimize outcomes and minimize complications.

Surgical vs. Nonsurgical Considerations

A traditional surgical facelift can turn back the clock on your appearance in several different ways. These are some benefits of surgical facelifts:

They tighten facial muscles. The underlying structures of your face tend to weaken and sag with age. Before repairing the loose skin, your plastic surgeon will tighten this underlying structure into a better configuration. This puts less tension on your skin, enabling the result of your facelift to last longer.

They repair loose skin. Your plastic surgeon can trim and tighten your sagging skin to ensure a more youthful and natural look. However, your surgeon must ensure that your skin is not drawn too tight, as that this can result in a "pulled" appearance.

They improve facial contours. If you opt for a mid facelift, this will result in a smoother look to the cheeks and lower eyelids. A lower facelift, on the other hand, results in a more attractive jawline contour, getting rid of jowls and smoothing out the neck area.

The results are lasting. The effects of a surgical facelift can last for up to ten years.

Here are some of the benefits of nonsurgical facelifts:

- **They are more cost-effective—at least in the near term.** If money is an issue, a nonsurgical facelift can offer an affordable value.

- **There is no serious pain involved.** With a nonsurgical facelift, there is minimal discomfort and pain experienced by the patient throughout the treatment.

- **The procedure time is short.** With a nonsurgical facelift, there is no anesthesia or other medication involved, and so these procedures can be completed within an hour. However, each patient is different, and so the procedure time may vary.

- **They result in a naturally rejuvenated look.** In a nonsurgical facelift, the skin is not cut or pulled tight, but is usually plumped and volumized, which can give the facial features and skin a youthful look.

- **The recovery time is minimal.** With nonsurgical facelifts, there is minimum time needed for the patient to take off work or other necessary activities and tasks. The recovery time is minimal, as opposed to a traditional surgical facelift. In fact, after a nonsurgical facelift, you can be back at work in no time!

- **The aftercare is also minimal.** Also, the aftercare involved following a nonsurgical facelift is minimal. Discomfort is relatively short-lived and can be managed with over-the-counter medication.

Perhaps the nonsurgical option sounds too good to be true—and sometimes surgery is absolutely necessary to achieve your objectives. This is why it's imperative to choose a board-certified plastic surgeon in order to be assured of an honest answer.

Nonsurgical Facial Tightening Procedures

elōs "Sublative" Skin Rejuvenation: Compared to other resurfacing treatments, which commonly use more aggressive ablative lasers requiring a longer recovery time, the sublative skin rejuvenation technology uniquely and precisely penetrates the skin. It then applies radio frequency (RF) energy directly (and deeper) into the dermal layers of the skin to stimulate collagen production while tightening elastic fibers without disrupting the superficial epidermal cells. This energy can be used on any skin color or tone without the worry of bleaching the skin pigment.

This rejuvenation procedure has been proven to be a safe, effective, and efficient treatment that provides yet another way for patients to achieve and maintain younger-looking skin.

elōs "Sublime" Skin Rejuvenation: Many patients are now opting to use this innovation for their "quick fix" or "lunchtime treatment" skin rejuvenation solution because there is no downtime and it can usually be completed in less than an hour.

Sublime technology is known by the nickname "Red Carpet Facelift" because of the immediate lifting, plumping, and tightening effects without downtime. The long-term benefits of enhanced tone and lift improve all aspects of the signs of aging.

This procedure features the revolutionary elōs combination of bi-polar radio frequency and infrared light energies to precisely heat the dermal tissue within the targeted treatment area. The energy stimulates collagen production and contracts elastin fibrils, resulting in an immediate lift with long-term production of collagen.

Wrinkle appearance is reduced, subtle lifting is achieved, and the skin's texture improved by becoming tighter, smoother, more vibrant, and toned. All this without enduring any downtime!

CO_2RE Fractionated Skin Rejuvenation: "Fractional" therapy refers to the pixilated distribution of laser light. Using a CO_2 laser, fractionated treatment allows for smaller thermal injuries than with fully ablative resurfacing. This also results in shorter downtime and fewer complications.

As opposed to older, traditional CO_2 lasers, CO_2RE is versatile, giving plastic surgeons the ability to treat both superficial and deep skin layers simultaneously, while maintaining precise control.

This noninvasive treatment usually allows patients to achieve light, moderate, and even deep wrinkle reduction, as well as skin resurfacing and scar reduction—often in a single session.

CO_2RE Ablative: With this facial resurfacing treatment, 100 percent of the epidermal layer of skin is removed. This treatment encourages the production of collagen in the skin cells to provide healthy, glowing skin.

Uniquely, the CO_2RE laser can be precisely adjusted at different levels, various intensities, and using different patterns to target the desired dermal levels of the skin, providing the exact rejuvenation level desired. In one session, this ablative procedure commonly eliminates wrinkles, scars, and sun damage.

ThermiSmooth: Over the years, our skin starts to lose collagen, elasticity, and plumpness. ThermiSmooth uses a thermal camera along with radiofrequency energy with a temperature-controlled instrument, which helps to smooth out the skin, usually providing patients with glowing results.

Your surgeon is able to select a precise temperature for stimulating the cells that firm and restore skin, and the ThermiSmooth system will flutter off and on to maintain that temperature. The instrument will indicate the precise temperature the skin has actually reached, so that there is no damage to the surrounding skin cells and tissue.

The ThermiSmooth treatment can address multiple areas to help with skin rejuvenation, which include forehead, eyes, cheeks, mouth, and neck. Many patients claim it feels like a warm massage.

One of its many benefits is that there is no downtime associated with this treatment. Recovery is immediate. You may be pink in the treated area for up to an hour and your skin may feel tighter, but that is temporary.

A series of ThermiSmooth sessions can restore radiance, propel collagen production, and shrink those crepey areas back into plump, radiant, healthy-looking skin of any color.

CO_2, IPL, and VBeam Lasers: More and more patients are deciding to use laser treatment therapy as it is less invasive than traditional surgical procedures.

CO_2 lasers have been around for decades and benefit patients with skin tightening and facial rejuvenation. They help to eliminate wrinkles, fine lines, and scarring and provide patients with smooth, glowing skin. The laser damages the deep layers of the skin, which stimulates the body's natural healing process, creating new, vibrant skin tissue.

The recovery from CO_2 laser treatment typically lasts around two weeks. Most patients find the treatment itself to be quick, with minimal discomfort.

The **IPL photofacial** is an intense pulsed-light procedure. The light penetrates deep into the skin, then the photo-rejuvenation causes the blood vessels and collagen to constrict. This reduces redness and fine lines. This treatment can improve sun damage, wrinkles, skin pigmentation, and more.

Many patients are choosing to undergo this laser treatment because it's noninvasive and doesn't cause any damage to the outer layer of skin. With the IPL, you typically can resume daily activities immediately. It is important to avoid direct sunlight for a few weeks and to wear sunscreen in order for the skin to heal properly, with results lasting longer.

The **Vbeam laser** is a pulsed dye laser with dual wavelengths and dual cooling, which can provide a better treatment procedure for individuals. The pulsed dye laser delivers intense but gentle light into targeted areas of the skin. The light is then absorbed by blood vessels or melanin in the skin.

This treatment helps mainly with spider veins and pigmented lesions of the skin, but can also treat rosacea, scars, stretch marks, warts, wrinkles, and vascular lesions. Most people return to their daily routine immediately, as there is no downtime associated with this treatment.

Yuni's Laser Story

For the majority of Yuni's life, she was plagued by cystic acne.

> I did isotretinoin treatments, and once I was rid of the cystic acne, my physician told me my next and best course of action regarding scars was to have my face laser resurfaced. My acne scars were deep, and in all honesty, I was afraid that I was going to grow up to look like Edward James Olmos, so I was determined to prevent that as best I could.

Yuni was anxious to discuss her treatment with a CO_2 laser.

> I've had it done two times. The first time was my entire face, the second time was just my cheeks. Laser treatment is wild. The procedure is fast, the recovery time short, and then there is a long period of stasis and then suddenly...a new face.

> Not painful, but there is pressure. There are various settings to the laser, so how deep it's going changes the way that it feels on the face. The areas that could be felt the most were around my hairline, around the lips, and along the jaw. After the fact, the skin bleeds some and starts to swell, it feels like an intense sunburn.

You only know your skin is there because you can feel your blood pulse in your cheeks.

She is very open about her recovery period.

The recovery is frightening. You just look scary; there is no polite way around it. I was aware of that, so it didn't come as too much of a surprise. Still, if you were to ask my husband and children today, they would tell you that for about three days after, they were afraid to look at me.

Then it's almost like a Bugs Bunny cartoon: the face just kind of crackles off and then this new, pink skin, which has never seen the light of day, is there, and it's smooth and glowy and incredibly fragile. That new skin needs to be kept out of the sun for some time.

Yuni's joy about her results is readily apparent.

Oh my goodness, I feel so cute now. My skin is so soft, so smooth. The skin is firmer, and I look rested. I look better than I did as a teenager, and now my friends think I'm aging backward.

I used to spend at least a good hour, maybe two, on my morning routine, layering various creams, balms, and cosmetics to smooth out my skin texture and even out my skin tone. Now it takes me about ten minutes to get myself together in the morning.

Less Invasive Neck Lift Options

Z-Plasty Neck Lift: This method is an alternative to the traditional neck lift. Z-Plasty is beneficial for candidates who have redundant skin, unwanted neck fat, and some skin creases. The procedure rearranges the tissue in the neck at two different angles. This approach has the ability to completely rejuvenate sagging skin in the neck into a more defined, natural-looking profile. It can be performed with local anesthesia, so no heavy sedation is required.

Neck Liposuction and Injectable RF: This technique is a combination of liposuction and Thermi Injectable Radiofrequency. First, the liposuction is done through small incisions made around the earlobe and chin/neck crease. Then the RF is used to help melt the residual fat, while contouring the loose skin for a defined neck profile. Ideal candidates for this method have good skin elasticity with isolated superficial fat.

Kybella: It's an injectable designed for dissolving fat under the chin. This procedure is extremely convenient for patients since it is minimally invasive, performed in-office, and does not require anesthesia. For the best results, the treatment often requires three to four sessions to dissolve diet-resistant fat.

The injections are designed to remove layers of fat without harming the underlying neck structures. The only limitation of this method is that skin laxity is not affected.

The Beauty of Injectables & Dermal Fillers

Injectables such as Botox and dermal fillers are cosmetic procedures to treat wrinkles and signs of aging. They are both minimally invasive and can provide long-lasting results. However, that's where their similarities end. These two injectables differ in terms of uses, efficacy, side effects, and of course, cost. Knowing the differences will help you choose which one is best for your needs.

Botox is the brand name for botulinum toxin, a neuromodulator produced by the bacterium *Clostridium botulinum*. Less commonly known brand names for botulinum toxin are Dysport and Jeuveau.

Botox prevents your nerves from transmitting signals to your muscles. This allows your muscles to relax so that they do not form fine lines and wrinkles.

Professionals inject Botox to target the muscles responsible for facial expression. As a result, it can address the "crows' feet" in the corners of the eyes, the frown lines (or "11s") between the eyebrows, and the lines on the forehead.

You will see the effects of Botox setting in as early as one to three days and experience the full effects in ten to fourteen days post-procedure. These results should last for three to six months. However, unlike fillers, Botox is not reversible.

FYI: Botox has other uses besides treating wrinkles on the face. It can alleviate other medical conditions including migraines, bruxism (teeth grinding), and hyperhidrosis (excess sweating) in the armpits.

Dysport: Many people are looking for a Botox treatment that targets specific areas and gives them natural-looking results. The "frozen look" is a big concern for people interested in neuromodulators. Dysport has been created to enable freedom to make facial expressions.

The differences lie in the potency of trace proteins, which can make one more effective than the other. This is why it is essential to have a board-certified plastic surgeon evaluate you with their specialized expertise.

Dysport helps to treat moderate to severe frown lines that appear between the eyebrows. It does this by reducing the specific muscle activity in the area. Since frown lines are caused by repeated muscle movements and contractions, along with wrinkles, they can appear early in life, even in someone in their twenties.

To treat the area, the injection is made into five different points between and above the eyebrows. Since this treatment is targeted specifically between the brows, this leaves the rest of your face to move freely. It's a quick treatment that can be done in as little as ten minutes, leaving you free to go about your day.

Jeuveau® is a prescription medication that prevents your nerves from telling your facial muscles to flex, temporarily smoothing moderate to severe lines between the brows. Some patients may experience better results with Jeuveau than Botox or Dysport. This is yet another reason to visit a plastic surgery practice for a careful, in-depth examination.

Jeuveau is perhaps best known for its ability to treat frown lines (glabellar lines). Two separate trials reported by the FDA found that 67 percent and 71 percent of people saw significant improvements after receiving these injections.

Dermal fillers are composed of a variety of materials. The most frequently used injectable fillers are the hyaluronic acid-based dermal fillers with brand names such as JUVÉDERM, Restylane, Radiesse, and Sculptra.

Hyaluronic acid is a naturally occurring sugar molecule that is a key component of the structural matrix that holds all the cells in your skin together. It forms a gel-like matrix by cross-linking large numbers of hyaluronic acid subunits with water and forms highly organized proteoglycan (or protein and sugar) complexes with the most abundant protein in our body: collagen.

In addition to its structural role, hyaluronic acid performs many crucial functions, some of which include tissue regeneration, wound healing, induction of collagen formation, and free radical scavenging. As we age, the amount of hyaluronic acid present in our skin, especially the top layer of our skin known as the epidermis, decreases dramatically.

JUVÉDERM® is a leader in the field of dermal fillers—produced by the same company that manufactures Botox—and offers five products to meet different specific needs.

This product line enables you to add volume to plump lips, smooth lines, contour cheeks, or shape the chin. Each product in the JUVÉDERM line features different bonding and concentrations of hyaluronic acid, each tailored to target specific problems when injected into different areas and depths.

During a procedure, your surgeon or nurse typically uses a pen to mark the areas to be treated. He/she will then inject a JUVÉDERM substance into the target area. They will also lightly massage the area to ensure an even distribution and reduce the chance of swelling.

The entire procedure usually takes between fifteen and sixty minutes, depending on the area or areas treated. JUVÉDERM injectables also contain a small amount of pain-reducing lidocaine to help minimize any pain or discomfort. Recovery time is minimal, and most patients notice the effects of JUVÉDERM right away, or soon after the swelling reduces. Results typically last between six months and two years, depending upon which JUVÉDERM product was used.

Restylane® is another injectable filler that helps smooth out fine lines, wrinkles, and folds on the face. It can also provide lip augmentation by adding plumpness to the lips and face, often creating a smooth, younger appearance.

Restylane is a fairly easy cosmetic procedure and can be performed right in a doctor's office without incisions. It's usually done with local anesthesia to minimize any discomfort you might experience.

Depending on how much work you're having done and the procedure itself, Restylane injections can take anywhere from a few minutes to half an hour.

Healing time will vary with each person and depends on how many injections you received and where. You can expect some redness, swelling, or bruising that might take a week or so to fully resolve. You should also limit your sun exposure afterward to prevent added swelling or bruising.

Full results are usually seen within a week after the procedure, but you will also see immediate effects since the products add volume when injected.

Restylane injections aren't permanent fillers, so if you want to maintain results, you'll need more rounds of injections. Depending on the kind of Restylane you received, the fillers last anywhere between six and eighteen months.

Radiesse® is another dermal filler that treats wrinkles and skin folds. It can increase the volume in areas of the face that can sag over time due to aging. This filler is also approved to treat volume loss in the backs of hands and is often useful for treating signs of aging around the mouth and chin.

Injections tend to cause a momentary pinching sensation. Many Radiesse providers may use the newer Radiesse + formulation, which includes a small amount of lidocaine present in the syringe to quell any discomfort.

Conclusion: Radiesse is a substance similar to ground-up bone, whereas Juvéderm and Restylane are smooth gels which are like a normal skin substance. Some plastic surgeons may prefer Juvéderm and Restylane to Radiesse because these fillers can be quickly and easily dissolved. Having said this, all three dermal fillers have proven effective in skin rejuvenation.

Sculptra® is helpful in restoring smooth skin. Collagen is the main protein responsible for keeping the skin looking young, as well as elastic, and

Sculptra is known as one of the longest-lasting fillers available. It has the ability to help the body create new collagen in order to correct wrinkles and folds of any depth.

There is no downtime associated with Sculptra, as most patients can return to their normal daily activities immediately after the treatment. Common side effects are swelling, bruising, and tenderness, which should resolve within a week.

To achieve the best results from the Sculptra aesthetic treatment, it is important to massage the area to help stimulate the collagen. The benefits from the treatment have been shown to last for up to two years in most patients.

Skin Rejuvenation

Is it really possible to recapture youthful, glowing skin? I suppose we can ask **Jennifer Garner**. Just look at that superb, glowing skin she displays in commercials. At fifty, her skin looks like that of someone in their twenties.

In an interview with *Shape* magazine, Jennifer stated, "I've focused on having the best possible skin that I can for my entire adult life. Because if my skin looks good, then I really don't care about makeup or hair."

Apparently, Jennifer has always been a big proponent of using retinol in her beauty routine. In a recent Instagram post, the actress shared her love for Neutrogena Rapid Wrinkle Repair Retinol Pro+ .5% Power Serum, which you can buy at Walmart for just twenty-nine dollars. The serum helps reduce fine lines and wrinkles for a youthful glow.

Unfortunately, most women are not endowed with Jennifer Garner's pristine skin or her resources—which are obviously spent on beauty services and products well beyond Walmart. But, fortunately, there are other skin rejuvenation avenues available to consumers and plastic surgery patients.

Microdermabrasion and **chemical peels** have proven effective in skin rejuvenation for many years. Microdermabrasion removes much of the top layer of skin in the epidermis, while chemical peels drive antioxidants into the living part of the skin, the dermis.

Basically, microdermabrasion is "mechanical" exfoliation, while chemical peels are chemical exfoliation. Selected on the basis of your skin type, there are also a variety of chemical peels for acne, pigmentation, and anti-aging.

Since human skin typically regenerates at approximately thirty-day intervals, microdermabrasion is temporary and needs to be repeated at average intervals of two to four weeks for continued improvement.

Depending on your skin, the strength of the chemical peel, and your tolerance of the procedure, the usual waiting period is two to four weeks between treatments. New skin regrowth may take from ten to fourteen days after a peel; thus, your face may be very red, sensitive, and dry until it has time to heal.

Topical Medications: Only highly trained medical staff should help you select medical-grade products that will enhance your skin's appearance.

Tretinoin (brand names Retin-A, Avita, Renova): Medical-grade Tretinoin requires a licensed physician to prescribe it in varying concentrations. Tretinoin has a long track record of being cost-efficient, effective, and a reliable method for skin collagen production, resulting in a more youthful skin look. This medication can improve skin texture when used regularly.

Hydroquinones: Often referred to as skin bleaching agents, higher concentrations (greater than 2 percent) are once again only available with a prescription from a licensed physician. Hydroquinones have a long track record of success for lightening those pigment irregularities often referred to as sun spots, liver spots, age spots, or freckles. Hydroquinone works by decreasing the amount of pigment produced by the melanocytes (cells that produce melanin, which determines your skin tone).

By reducing melanin production, your skin will potentially become more evenly toned over time. On average, it takes about four weeks of regular use to start to see results and may take several months before you see full results.

Importance of a Qualified Aesthetician: Most plastic surgery practices have licensed aestheticians on staff. An aesthetician will evaluate your skin without makeup, revealing your true skin type. This allows them to recommend professional treatments and products appropriate for your skin type and your skin care needs.

A plastic surgeon's aesthetician can also perform medical-grade facials. These facials provide a clinical approach to treatment, generally with far greater benefits than available at a typical spa. Typically, an aesthetician teams with the plastic surgeon to create a customized treatment plan based upon a patient's skin type and needs.

Charlene has quite an interesting story regarding her "mask of pregnancy." These are brownish blotches on the skin around the eyes, nose, and cheeks that are common in pregnancy, thus this nickname. (The official names for this condition are chloasma or melasma.)

"I gave birth to twins a couple months after my twenty-third birthday," says Charlene. "Over the years, I developed the 'mask of pregnancy.' I had no idea what that was until I was in a dressing room surrounded by mirrors and perfect lighting. I had it so bad, I broke down in tears and never wanted to see myself again."

Charlene explains she discovered an aesthetician who put her on the right track. "Then I found Alicia, who was working at a plastic surgery practice. She recommended dermabrasion, and I cannot tell you how much that helped me."

For many years, Charlene has continued with this aesthetician whenever the need arises. "Now it's wrinkles and sun spots, but I never have to worry about these things because Alicia knows just what I need, and she keeps a smile on my face."

Dr. Hardesty: In the last ten years, new and more effective noninvasive and minimally invasive treatments, and minimal incision procedures, have continued to evolve to offer patients more options for cosmetic improvement with minimal downtime. For example, when these nonsurgical enhancements are combined with short-scar surgical procedures, the results can be dramatic.

Every patient is unique, and multiple modalities/options can be required to provide the latest technologies to reach the patient's goals.

Dr. Polakof: Nonsurgical facial procedures are not only good options in some cases but can save time and money. However, regardless of which treatment option you ultimately choose, it's important to find a trained, skilled provider with extensive experience performing cosmetic injections.

Additionally, when searching for facial rejuvenation, a great price is no substitute for receiving the best possible care and excellent, long-lasting aesthetic results.

CHAPTER 14

BODY CONTOURING

"Body love is more than acceptance of self or the acceptance
of the body. Body love is about self-worth in general. It's more than
our physical appearance."

—Mary Lambert

Women often struggle in their relationships with their bodies, and their tummies are no exception! Genetics, aging, body shape, hormones, diet, and pregnancies all factor into the shape of a woman's body.

The gold standard for abdominal body contouring has always been liposuction and/or a tummy tuck. Whether you need one or both depends on your goals and on your anatomy.

 **Liposuction**, sometimes referred to as "lipo" by patients, slims and reshapes specific areas of the body by removing excess fat deposits and improving your body contours and proportion. A plastic surgeon can utilize liposuction to treat a wide variety of areas, including your abdomen, waist, thighs, hips, buttocks,

ankles, and upper arms. Fat can even be removed in facial areas such the neck, cheeks, and chin. It's also important to understand that liposuction offers no value in attempting to treat obesity or cellulite.

Although liposuction is not a technically difficult procedure, it requires thoughtful planning and a surgeon's artistic eye to achieve aesthetically pleasing postoperative results. The goal of the liposuction surgeon is to remove "target" fat, leaving the desired body contour and smooth transitions between suctioned and non-suctioned areas.

Janie from Georgia provides some realistic goals for having liposuction. "I'm not overweight, I've never been overweight, but I have always had fat in very unwelcome places. A common misconception is that liposuction is for weight loss—it isn't. It's more for when you're close to or at your ideal weight, but you need to sculpt out the shape you want to be."

Like many women, Janie's challenge was common. "My trouble area has always been the 'love handle' region. To add insult to injury, I have really high hip bones, so I've always felt like—next to my long, skinny legs and my long slender arms, my stomach had always looked like a tire."

What surprised Janie was the integrity of her surgeon.

> My doctor explained everything that would happen step by step during the procedure and what to expect for recovery. He also carefully laid out that, due to some of the more difficult to reach pockets of fat that I have on my body, I will likely need a follow-up procedure in about twelve weeks. When you have a physician that is completely honest like that, there's truly nothing like it. I wasn't expecting perfection from this procedure, more like just improvement. Currently, I'm in my third week post-op, and it feels like my procedure was performed months before. I am so excited to watch my body continue to change for the better.

Janie is so very correct. There are complications with liposuction that can occur at the hands of an unskilled or inexperienced surgeon—so choose wisely. Risks include contour irregularities where your skin will appear bumpy or wavy, which can be permanent. If the cannula penetrates too deeply, it can puncture an internal organ, or pieces of loosened fat may break away and become trapped in a blood vessel or gather in the lungs.

Advanced Methods of Liposculpture

There are a number of liposculpture methods. Once your plastic surgeon completes a thorough examination to determine the quantity of fat that needs to be removed and inspects your skin's elasticity, he or she will describe the most suitable options.

Tumescent Liposuction: This treatment utilizes local anesthesia, normal saline, and dilute epinephrine (to minimize blood loss), which is injected prior to liposculpture. This combination helps cause the blood vessels to constrict and lessens the postoperative pain.

Suction-Assisted Liposuction: This is the traditional form of liposuction, using a thin tubular cannula which draws out the unwanted fatty deposits utilizing a surgical vacuum.

Power-Assisted Liposuction: This technology utilizes the traditional suction-assisted form of liposuction, and in addition, initiates tiny but rapid vibrations to break up fat cells so that they can be suctioned more effectively.

Ultrasound-Assisted Liposuction: This method adds energy through a hand piece which helps to melt the fat and disrupts fibrous tissue while loosening the fat connections. Then standard suction-assisted liposuction follows to remove the disrupted tissue and fat.

Laser-Assisted Liposuction: This is a newer technology that utilizes a laser beam in conjunction with standard-assisted liposuction to help disrupt the fat cells and make fat removal more efficient.

Dr. Polakof: I wish to convey that Dr. Hardesty has developed a new pre-/postoperative technology he named the T-U-L-I-P liposculpture protocol. The T represents tumescent fluid, which he injects prior to the procedure to control postoperative pain; U stands for ultrasonic liposuction, which utilizes sonic waves to break up fibrous and scar tissues, dissolving fat cells; L relates to his liposculpture technique to remove and sculpt fat tissue; I refers to investing in garments which compress the skin against the muscle to form the body to the new sculpted contour; and P designates postoperative use of nonsurgical **VellaShape III,** which delivers radio frequency energy and external gentle suction to shrink the skin and improve the texture.

Dr. Hardesty has trained other plastic surgeons in this unique technique; thus it may be available elsewhere.

In terms of recovery from a liposuction procedure, patients typically return to daily activities and non-strenuous work within a few days. Improvements are often seen immediately, but it may take a few months to obtain the final results as the skin contours to the new shape.

Tucking Your Tummy

 She's a middle-aged woman from Kansas, and we'll call her Dorothy. Her decision to have a tummy tuck (known as abdominoplasty) is one many women can identify with.

Over the years, I had lost sight of whose gigantic panties I was folding in the laundry...they were mine. I made jokes about my size, claiming it was just another growing stage. In an attempt to disguise my size, I wore tent dresses, but in my white sundress I looked like a giant lemon meringue pie. I knew I had to do something to stop my body's fat expansion plans or I was going to spend the rest of my life uncomfortable and unhealthy.

Dorothy's first step to turn this around was her visit to a dietician.

She told me to regard fast food as FAT food and to avoid it at all costs. Daily walks and exercise became a necessity, just as important as eating and sleeping. Slowly my energy level began to increase, my weight began to decrease, but the skin that had held all my weight seemed to be growing. Finally, one day while walking with a friend, I told her about my frustration, and she revealed that three pregnancies had left her with a kangaroo pouch. The elasticity in her skin had not retracted back to its original shape, but all was not lost. She had a tummy tuck and suggested I look into one as well.

I spent that night on the internet and found a board-certified plastic surgeon in my area. At my appointment, I had the opportunity to see photos of patients for whom the surgeon had performed this procedure. All of my questions were answered in-depth and, after my preoperative appointment I was on my way to being sculpted.

Dorothy fondly recalls her recovery experience.

I spent the first night after surgery resting comfortably at the surgical center. This had been a deciding factor in choosing my surgeon, as fellow tummy tuck warriors had advised me of the importance of an overnight stay at the surgical center. Two tiny drains, whom I affectionately named "Big Gulp" and "Slim Fast," removed excess fluid from my tummy for a week. I was back to work in a week, and at two weeks started throwing away my elastic waist pants. By six weeks, I had multiple wardrobe choices.

Dorothy concludes by celebrating her victory. "I enjoy my body and the good health it provides me. There is a scar that hides just below my panty line, but I consider it more of a souvenir from a battle I once won."

Many women after pregnancy can't get rid of the "mommy bump," loose skin, or stretch marks despite returning to their pre-pregnancy weight. Both men and women who have tried to lose stubborn diet-resistant belly fat through exercise and diet often become discouraged and frustrated by the challenge. And after bariatric surgery, a person is left with excess skin which doesn't shrink.

A tummy tuck, medically referred to as abdominoplasty, is a treatment option to help get rid of this excess skin and fat. Additionally, plastic surgeons can perform variations of a tummy tuck, which can include liposuction of the flanks where "muffin top" fat accumulation occurs.

Customizing Your Figure

Depending on your desired aesthetic goals, as well as the amount and location of excess skin and fatty tissue, tummy tuck techniques will vary. Usually, a plastic surgeon will make the incision as low on the abdomen as possible, which is designed to be hidden by a bathing suit or panties.

This incision allows the removal of the excess fat and skin tissue as well as tightening the separated muscles, permanently removing unwanted fat and loose skin. Adding liposuction of the flanks will redrape and tightly stretch the skin to fit the body's new and natural contours.

Mini Abdominoplasty: This is ideal for those who are in good shape but have some general isolated laxity and diet-resistant specific fat of the lower abdomen. A single short incision is usually made just above the pubic area. In contrast to other tummy tuck procedures, there is no incision around the belly button (umbilicus). A mini tummy tuck often includes liposuction as well as tightening the muscles to create an attractive body contour.

Extended Abdominoplasty: If one has significant excess skin and fat around the hips and love handles area, in addition to a standard tuck, this technique removes skin and fat over the frontal hip area and tightens the layers above the hips.

Fleur De Lis Abdominoplasty: This type of tummy tuck is employed for individuals with significant weight loss or those with significant excess horizontal, mid, and upper abdominal fat and skin. It's similar to an extended abdominoplasty with an added vertical component incision allowing direct removal of excess tissue, fat, and skin in the central and upper abdomen.

Note: There is a resultant vertical scar. However, this is considered a small trade-off for getting permanently rid of the significant accumulation of upper, mid, and lower abdominal fat rolls and the redundant loose skin.

Reverse Abdominoplasty: This option is infrequently used except for isolated upper abdominal excess fat and loose skin. The incision is made in the breast crease, and the excess skin and fat is pulled up and resected.

The recovery period usually lasts four to seven days before returning to normal daily activities. A non-narcotic pain pump (installation of constant local anesthesia for the first three days after surgery) is usually included with tummy tucks. This reduces pain and the need for pain pills after surgery.

Some plastic surgery practices also provide an anti-scar program after the incisions are healed. When performed by a board-certified plastic surgeon, tummy tuck surgery results are usually quite flattering and last for many years.

Additional Body-Sculpting and Contouring Procedures

Brazilian Buttock Lift

 Known for her appealing curves and shapely butt, Kim Kardashian is considered one of the pioneers on this turf. However, she has always denied allegations that she has butt implants, even going to the extent of revealing x-ray photos of her butt.

Note: While silicone butt implants would clearly appear on an x-ray, a Brazilian buttock lift wouldn't, because it involves the use of a patient's own body fat. It is reported that over forty thousand BBLs were performed in a single year. Women simply want the butt appearance of a Kim Kardashian or Jennifer Lopez.

A Brazilian buttock lift, also known as buttock augmentation, is a procedure that is designed to help women obtain an uplifted and shapelier buttock. Basically, it is performed by taking "unwanted" body fat, and after purification, injecting it into the buttocks. Precise liposculpture is performed around the areas of the buttock to make it shapelier.

One option is to utilize silicone implants, which are placed into the natural buttock crease, which lift and shape the buttocks for a desired look.

Typically, patients are given anti-swelling and anti-bruising medication preoperatively. However, some bruising and swelling is expected after the procedure. Most patients can return to daily activities within a few days, and full exercise is allowed after six weeks.

What Seven Women Who Had a Brazilian Buttock Lift Would Have Done Differently

In interviews conducted by Real Self, seven women who underwent a BBL procedure were asked what they would do differently.

I would have worn my compression garment much longer. I feel if I had worn it longer, it would have helped with the inflammation.
—**Kai**, 39, Raleigh, NC

I would have taken longer to recover. There is no need to be Superwoman after surgery, but I went and walked around the South Beach shopping area. I traveled back home five days post-op and went back to work seven days post-op. I was okay, but in hindsight, I would give myself more time to recover.
—**Megan**, 37, Denver

If I could go back, I would have lost more weight prior to surgery. Because I was so heavy going in, even with my doctor taking the maximum amount of fat that he could take out, I was still left with a lot that I needed to lose. And I didn't want to lose my reinjected fat cells, so I was just torn between losing my gut or my butt.
—**Suzy**, 34, Minneapolis

I would have never done my first BBL surgery—that was by far the biggest mistake I have ever made, and to this day I am still trying to fix it. For the first surgery, the doctor totally destroyed the skin on my butt cheeks—some areas are sunken, some lumpy, and my scars are very thick. It was bad. I originally wanted to go to another doctor, and I should have done what I wanted from the beginning. By trying to go a little cheaper, I did myself no favors and have spent over $36,000 just hoping to fix it. I'm going to need to do another BBL, so that's even more money.
—**Missginger**, 29, Kennewick, WA

I wish I hadn't looked for a surgeon based on how much I wanted to pay. I should have focused on saving for longer, then going to the best doctor in my city. My results aren't terrible, but I feel like they could be so much better. My butt looks lumpier than it did before surgery—like I have cellulite in new places—and my doctor just kind of cut off communication after my follow-up appointments. —**Jane**, 27, Atlanta

I would have definitely chosen a different surgeon. The doctor who performed my BBL didn't actually enjoy performing the surgery and only did a few of them per year. I chose him because my coworker and her friends highly recommended him—however, they had chosen him for different procedures. If I were under the knife again for a second BBL, I would ensure a detailed investigation of the area surgeons and choose one who has a lot of BBL experience. —**Nickie**, 47, Virginia Beach, Virginia

I would not have done anything differently. I had done a lot of research before deciding to go ahead with the procedure and knew what I was getting into. My doctor was very good and prioritized safety. I wasn't willing to travel because of the long recovery involved and the inability to sit, but I was very happy with the doctor I chose. Since my healing and final results, however, I've decided to go for a second round of surgery to give more projection in the upper part of my bum and accentuate the hourglass shape. —**Chloe**, 25, Canberra, Australia

Body Lift

Dramatic weight loss, aging skin, major weight fluctuations, and bariatric surgery can result in non-elastic skin that sags. A body lift procedure can create a more slender, athletic, and firm shape with one circular incision located at the lower hip area that is easily hidden by normal clothes or swimwear.

A plastic surgeon experienced and skilled in this procedure can address multiple areas in one surgical session, which includes the abdomen, hips, thighs, and buttock concurrently.

Can you imagine your thighs not touching each other? Thick, bulging inner and outer thighs with saggy, loose, stretched skin can preclude wearing certain clothes and even interfere with walking and exercise. Common to all the thigh lifts is both liposuction and resection of excess skin and fat. The larger the resection of skin and fat, the longer the resultant healed incision will be. However, many plastic surgery practices provide a proven anti-scar program.

Arm Lift

 An increasing number of women are choosing to tighten the appearance of their arms with an arm lift procedure. These patients often feel that the excess skin on their arms is unflattering due to some amount of drooping or sagging. An arm lift procedure, also referred to as brachioplasty, is designed to reshape the arm by removing unwanted hanging, flapping skin and arm fat, resulting in a slenderer arm appearance.

Most patients can usually return to daily activities within a few days. There are aids to help in the healing process, such as compression garments that you may need to wear for six weeks.

Dr. Hardesty: During my career, the improvement of safety and predictable results have made great strides in body contouring, especially abdominoplasty (tummy tucks). Combining limited incisional surgery, minimal undermining, precise adjunct liposuction, postoperative pain reduction (via pain pumps), and the quilting suture technique have made this procedure much more predictable, safer, and with faster recovery times.

Dr. Polakof: In order to be confident that your tummy tuck surgeon can deliver the beautiful results you desire, you should ask to see a variety of before and after photos of former patients. This will give you a good idea as to the quality of work the surgeon achieves, and what you can expect from your tummy tuck procedure. Ask him or her to point out an example which best compares to their approach for your procedure.

You must feel very comfortable with your tummy tuck surgeon. He or she should make you feel relaxed throughout the entire process and be willing to spend as much time as needed to answer all of your questions.

CHAPTER 15

MOMMY MAKEOVER

"No one is in control of your happiness but you. Therefore, you have the power to change anything about yourself or your life that you want to change."

—Barbara de Angelis

 The goal of a **mommy makeover** is to restore the shape and appearance of a woman's body after childbearing. These physical unwanted changes can manifest themselves as a baby bump, smaller, deflated, droopy breasts, stretch marks, and diet-resistant fatty deposits. There are many areas of the body that can be addressed collectively, most commonly the breasts, abdomen, waist, genitalia, and buttocks.

Our first words of wisdom come from an article written by an anonymous woman who wanted other mothers to know about things she wished she had known before her mommy makeover.

Guilty as charged. As most moms do, I tend to put everyone else first. A lot of times, that is why women feel like they have lost their identities. It's hard to spend that much money on yourself, especially for aesthetic reasons. It seems okay to spend it on a car or a trip, but for some reason, the thought of spending that money on your body is frowned upon.

To some, that may seem vain or boastful. For me, it was about a self-confidence that I had yet to achieve, a love of self that I have longed for my entire life. When I look in the mirror, I like what I see now. When I feel good about myself—inside and out—I am a better woman, a better wife, and a better mom.

It is absolutely normal to feel guilty about spending money on a mommy makeover, and it is okay to finally put yourself first. It is the best money I have ever spent...just ask my family.

I'm a big girl now. Most mommy makeovers include lipo and a tummy tuck. Which probably means you will be lucky enough to wear a skin-tight crotchless compression garment. I, as most women, chose to wear panties over this outfit so I didn't feel as it all my "stuff" was being squished out. (Think of baboons...ewww, or don't.)

Now the tricky part here is the first couple of days after surgery. You will spend quite a bit of time on the toilet the first time you try to pee, similar to what it is like after giving birth. After a couple tries, it gets better. However, when you are taking pain medication and muscle relaxers on a regular basis, your mind may be fuzzy a bit.

Also, you will probably not poop for several days at first, so expect a good three to five days' worth of poop on your first time. With that being said, consider pulling your garment down for that endeavor.

Hello, Dolly! If you decide to get implants, please remember that objects may appear larger than they actually are. When I first took a glance at my new girls, I thought *Holy Mary, Mother of God, what have I done?* I looked like Dolly Parton, or for younger ones, Beth from Dog the Bounty Hunter. This is *not* your final look. Please don't freak out.

The swelling takes a while to go down and for the implants to "drop" into place. After about a week, your plastic surgeon will probably give you the go ahead to start massaging them. Massaging the implants will help them soften up and find their final resting place. Your significant other will love this, and surprisingly, so will you. I was shocked to find how much I actually liked touching my own breasts. It sounds perverted, I know, but if you are used to your "ladies" hanging out down by your belly, then you will see how nice it is to hold them, let go, and be fascinated that they no longer fall down so low anymore.

Phantom of the itch. I knew going into the tummy tuck part of the mommy makeover that my belly would be numb. It is a freaky and strange feeling. It is almost like you are rubbing on someone else's tummy. I had heard before about people who have had an arm or leg amputated and still felt the feeling of it being there, the phantom limb syndrome. I was not prepared for that with my belly. Every now and then, I will get an itch, go to scratch it, and realize it is where my belly is numb.

Sit. Stay. Good girl. Once again, most mommy makeovers include a tummy tuck. This is a huge procedure, and as most of you have surely read, it is a good idea to take off as much time as possible from your job.

Like most moms, I am an expert at multitasking. It was killing me to sit there and not do anything. The first three days or so, you have no choice; your body will not allow it. I will admit that

I probably did more than I should have. Looking back, I wish I had taken more advantage of the quiet time and rested and relaxed. Just take this time for yourself and give your body a chance to heal.

All aboard...the Bi-Polar Express. This is a *big* one. Having your body cut upon, stitched up, and hung up to dry is traumatic. Throw a few pain meds into the mix, and you will turn into an emotional tornado. I was known to go from ecstatic to tears in 6.9 seconds flat. Top that!!

Be aware that this will be an issue, and emotions will be crazy. Explain this to your loved ones and the people caring for you so they don't call the men in white coats with the straitjackets.

Let's get physical. Most people who are looking into plastic surgery are doing so because exercise has not been effective on certain areas of the body. There are only so many chest flies one can do before you realize they won't make your boobies stand up and say hello.

However, there are some who think this is the alternative to diet and exercise. If that is you, you're wrong. I truly believe my fitness level aided in my recovery time. And I know that I will have to work twice as hard to keep my new body looking tip-top.

The more active and healthy you are before surgery, the better your recovery will be. You will heal faster, feel better sooner, and be back to the gym before you know it. As you heal, stay away from processed and salty foods, soda, and fried foods. When your doctor says it's okay, get back into exercising and let your body lead the way. It will tell you what is too much and when to quit.

Don't be naïve: Do the research. When I decide to do something, I go full speed, headfirst. In this case, you need to know what you are getting into. When I began this journey, I had no idea that there was a difference between a board-certified plastic surgeon and a board-certified cosmetic surgeon.

Ask around; find people who have used him/her. The doctor will give you referrals, but let's face it—they are not stupid enough to give you someone who is unhappy with their work.

Be wary of the flashy salesman. Go with your gut and ask *lots* of questions. The good ones will sit with you and take as much time as needed.

Avoid the Debbie Downers. We all know one...the Debbie Downers, the buzzkills. And most of us will have to deal with a few after surgery. It is really hard when you feel that you don't have the support from your loved ones.

The choice to have a mommy makeover is strictly yours, and **hopefully you are doing this for you and only you**. I have had a few family members that I surprisingly haven't received support from. It is hurtful, especially since they saw me struggle with my weight and self-esteem issues for years.

As long as you know why you are doing this, that is all you need. For me, being able to look in the mirror, smile, and for the first time in my life, love what I see...well, that is priceless to me. And for those who can't see past the money or their opinions, they are missing out on watching someone they love transforming into the person they have always dreamed of being.

More About Mommy Makeovers

The best time to get a mommy makeover is after you are completely done having children and breastfeeding—and after you have tried to reach your goal weight. When you are within twenty pounds of your goal weight, and it is stable, then it is a good time to undergo a mommy makeover. Will you lose weight? Generally, yes, since with liposuction and tummy tuck procedures, you are likely to lose some weight from removing unwanted fat and loose skin. Additionally, it is very common to continue to lose weight after a mommy makeover. Why? Because once they see and feel the difference, it stimulates patients to start an exercise program, improve their diets, and embrace a healthy lifestyle.

What amount of pain can one expect? Patients will normally be quite sore for about three to four days. Most plastic surgery practices offer pain pumps to make patients feel more comfortable during their healing.

How long is the recovery period? If the mommy makeover includes a tummy tuck, most patients will need at least two weeks before returning to the majority of daily activities. If you have a more active job, you might need four to six weeks off work. One should also expect to refrain from exercising for at least eight weeks, with the exception of light walks.

How will you feel about your mommy makeover? Here are comments from three more patients.

> **Stacy**: I have been dealing with the pain and suffering of having very large breasts for years, as well as an unflattering waistline due to giving birth and getting older. So I made the decision to have a mommy makeover (breast reduction and tummy tuck) for my fiftieth birthday. I *love* my new body! I'm three months post-surgery, and I have already lost twenty pounds. This investment into a better me was the best decision of my life.

> **Theresa**: I had a tummy tuck and breast lift and feel very satisfied with the results. Pregnancy did a number on my breasts, and I had a bad scar on my lower abdomen that is now gone. I guess the words would be confidence and comfort.

Sandi: After having three children, I was not pleased with the appearance of my breasts or abdomen, nor the way my clothes were fitting. I had lost my self-esteem and wanted to look and feel younger. On the human side, I wanted a surgeon who was realistic, had a sense of humor and some religious convictions, because a prayer before the actual surgery is very comforting. My research paid off, and I had a tummy tuck as well as breast enhancement. My advice to others is to do your research and educate yourself about the procedure(s) you want to be done. Lastly, do it sooner than later, because you're not getting younger. You can't save time in a bottle.

Full or Mini Tummy Tuck for Mommy Makeover?

While liposuction is the gold standard for removing excess fat, it cannot address sagging skin or loose muscles, both of which are common in patients who have had children or gained and lost a significant amount of weight. However, a tummy tuck can improve all these conditions. There are two options when it comes to the tummy tuck: a full tummy tuck and a mini tummy tuck.

The ideal candidate for a mini tummy tuck only has loose skin below the belly button. This basically rules out most women who have given birth, gained weight, or gone through menopause. The incision line may be a bit longer for the full, but it is the procedure to deliver a lean, fit-looking contour to your entire abdomen.

Three Mommies with Makeovers

Kerri is a New Jersey woman whose makeover story will be familiar to many moms.

After having two big baby boys, I was left with sagging skin and breasts and a shifted sense of self. What I saw in the mirror no longer matched the person I was.

I have always been a very fit, athletic person, and I worked hard to lose the weight I'd gained during my pregnancies—but it became very clear to me that, despite exercise and strict dieting, I would never be able to truly see the results I was working so hard for.

After a good amount of research, Kerri chose a plastic surgeon and decided upon a tummy tuck with muscle repair, liposuction of the flanks, and a breast lift with moderate implants under the muscle.

The first two days, what I felt most was the muscle soreness in my chest and the tightness of my abdomen. I was unable to stand up straight and had to sleep on an incline, and getting up from a lying position was not fun. But I never experienced any sharp, excruciating pains. After two days, I was taking Tylenol exclusively when needed, and things were smooth.

In the long run, Kerri was overjoyed with her mommy makeover experience.

My results are extreme, both externally and internally. My mind is finally free of the constant personal critiques, and that is such a blessing in itself.

I would wholeheartedly recommend getting a mommy makeover to any mothers who are considering it. Your happiness and peace of mind outweigh the monetary cost of surgery, and the downtime during recovery is nothing compared to the time you'll get back from not always being caught up in your mind.

Victoria hails from Texas. After giving birth to three children, including a set of twins, she set a goal for herself: to drop sixty pounds. This was the number she needed to reach in order to be approved for a breast reduction.

> I was physically in pain from my large breasts. Finally, I ended up losing a total of eighty pounds, but was left with excess skin that made physical activity difficult. It also made it difficult to find clothes that fit, and I felt very insecure about that. Instead of flaunting my weight loss, I was still hiding under lots of clothes. So a breast reduction turned into a mommy makeover—and it was the best decision I have ever made for myself.

Victoria chose a Houston plastic surgeon and decided upon a tummy tuck and liposuction to the flanks, as well as the breast reduction she'd originally set her sights on.

Her recovery was pretty intense. It involved limited mobility and some pain for the first week. Victoria states that she was back to her normal self within six weeks and there were no complications. Most important, she was thrilled with her new body.

> I am very happy with my results. I went from a 32F bra to a 32C, and I lost seven pounds of excess skin with my tummy tuck. Now I can physically move in ways I couldn't for the past ten years, and I'm as active as I was in high school. It was the greatest gift I could give myself.

Anne from Florida has a different story, and it's a bit of a wake-up call. Her mommy makeover was comprised of a tummy tuck, liposuction of the flanks, and breast augmentation.

> I am about six and a half months post-op now, and I'd say it was definitely worth it. I have gained so much confidence and feel so beautiful again. However, if you asked me when I was two to three months post-op, it was such a roller coaster of emotions. No one tells you how to prepare for what your mind will go

through and how you will be emotionally challenged every day. There were days I'd just cry when I looked at myself, because I expected certain results right away, and I didn't get that. Some days, I couldn't even look at myself and wished I'd never had the surgery. It is definitely a process—a hard one on your body and a tough one mentally.

The final outcome is mostly good news for Anne, but it's a mix.

Now I am mostly happy with my overall appearance. It has motivated me to begin working out again, to maintain my twenty-four-inch waist and get back into shape. The only thing I am unhappy with is my tummy tuck scar. I would have quit smoking cigarettes sooner if I'd had the chance to. From the time I first contacted the coordinator for my surgery was only twenty days, and I quit smoking in ten days. At the pre-op appointment, my doctor said my chances of developing necrosis were significantly higher since I had just quit smoking. He asked if I would reschedule. I did not, and I developed necrosis on my tummy tuck incision.

It was not as bad as it could have been, but my scar is thicker in the center, where the necrosis was the worst. It is fading nicely on the sides, but I think the center part of the scar will always be visible.

In support of these patient comments, according to the American Society of Plastic Surgeons, mommy makeovers have become incredibly popular over the last decade. They enable women to have multiple aesthetic procedures in a single surgery—and the results generally enhance their self-esteem.

When is it be okay to have sex after a mommy makeover? Generally, you will need to abstain for the first two weeks following surgery, possibly longer if your surgery is more involved. If your heart rate or blood pressure become elevated (during sex or other exercise), that can cause internal bleeding at your surgical sites.

Your abdominal muscles will be sutured. Contracting them before they've had a chance to start healing could cause tearing, and strenuous activity could also cause your incision to reopen. Many actually report that sex is better following their surgery. This may be due to an enhanced self-image, but there is also an anatomical reason for this experience. Abdominoplasty tightens the tummy, but it also lifts the pubic region, which repositions the clitoris over the pubic bone. This more youthful position of the clitoris against the pubic bone allows for more direct pressure during intercourse, enhancing the experience.

Dr. Hardesty: Breast surgery is often a fundamental component of the mommy makeover. A breast implant is a safe, excellent method for restoring this lost volume from childbirth. However, pregnancy, breastfeeding, and age can also stretch out the skin and tissues on your breasts. This is why a straightforward breast augmentation is not always the solution. When you stand in front of the mirror, do your nipples still face forward? If not, you are probably going to be better served with a breast lift, either on its own or with a breast implant.

Dr. Polakof: Many women ask about the ideal age to have a mommy makeover. It's definitely better to engage in these multiple procedures when your childbearing years are behind you, since a future pregnancy can negatively affect the results from your mommy makeover. Also, you want to be mentally prepared for such an array of aesthetic procedures, as we have seen from patient comments in this chapter.

CHAPTER 16

BREAST ENHANCEMENT

"Beauty is enhancing what you have. Let yourself shine through."
—Janelle Monae

A study published in the *International Journal of Sexual Health* found that 70 percent of women are dissatisfied with their breasts. These feelings of inadequacy make breast augmentation the top cosmetic surgery performed in the United States. Every year, over 300,000 women have breast enhancement surgery.

The American Society of Plastic Surgeons has conducted many studies on breast enhancement. Their research has found that 98 percent of women undergoing breast augmentation surgery say the results met or exceeded their expectations. Other studies have shown that breast implants can help boost self-esteem, body image, and sexual satisfaction.

Having said this, we are quite familiar with patients who were not pleased with their breast enhancement procedures and will now discuss the reasons why a number of negative comments have been made.

Dangers and Risks of Implants

Dissatisfaction and emotional despondency largely arise from patient fear or experiences with implants, as well as risks involved. Some of these risks and concerns arose in 2017 with the discovery of a link between textured breast implants and anaplastic large cell lymphoma, a rare type of non-Hodgkins lymphoma, commonly referred to as BIA-ALCL. This led breast-implant manufacturer Allergan to recall a number of its products from the market. Breast implant illness (BII) refers to a series of systemic symptoms which include fatigue, joint pain, hair loss, headaches, rash, brain fog, and depression. It should be noted that there haven't yet been any major studies into the number of women with breast implants who develop BII, but there are too many reported cases not to take this seriously.

Let's turn to other risks of breast implants:

- Scar tissue that distorts the shape of the breast implant (capsular contracture)

- Breast pain

- Infection

- Changes in nipple and breast sensation (often only temporary)

- Implant leakage or rupture

Any of these five conditions could ultimately mandate additional surgery or removal of the implants. (It should be noted that implants with textured silicone and polyurethane outer shells seem to pose the highest risk, particularly in respect to BIA-ALCL.)

Saline vs. Silicone: Which Breast Implants Are Right for You?

Saline implants have an outer shell, made of silicone, which are filled with sterile salt water, whereas silicone gel-filled implants are silicone shells filled with a plastic gel (silicone). While many women say that silicone gel implants feel more like real breasts than saline, they can pose more of a risk if they leak.

Saline might be best for you if:

- You have a good amount of natural breast tissue.

- You don't like the idea of getting MRIs to monitor your breast implants.

- You want the least expensive implant option. On average, saline implants cost quite a bit less than silicone.

The FDA recommends that women with silicone implants get routine MRI scans every two to three years to monitor for possible ruptures.

Silicone could be preferable if:

- You want a more natural look. While a skilled plastic surgeon can achieve a natural look with saline implants, the "natural give" consistency of silicone gel implants helps them look even more natural inside the breast.

- You also want a totally natural-feeling breast. There is no denying that silicone gel implants feel more like natural breast tissue.

- You have very little natural breast tissue. Because silicone implants have a more viscous filling than saline, rippling and wrinkling is much less of an issue. Thus, even patients with minimal or thin breast tissue can enjoy a natural look.

FDA Strengthens Breast-Implant Safety Requirements

The good news is that, whichever type of implant patients now choose, in October of 2021, the FDA took several new actions to strengthen breast-implant risk communication and help those who are considering breast implants make informed decisions. In the biggest shift, plastic surgeons and other health professionals who work with the implants must give their patients a checklist detailing possible side effects, such as scarring, pain, rupture, and even a rare form of cancer. The checklist also explains that breast implants may require repeat surgeries, and they should not be considered lifelong devices.

Note: Both saline and silicone breast implants are currently considered safe for breast augmentation and breast reconstruction. Research on the safety and effectiveness of both types of implants is ongoing.

Patient Satisfaction Continues to Be Strong

A study in the *Plastic and Reconstructive Surgery Journal* revealed that women who had breast enhancement surgery reported increased satisfaction with the appearance of their breasts and a greater sense of psychosocial and sexual well-being after the surgery.

Aysha, aged thirty, expressed that after breastfeeding, her confidence had been negatively affected.

My breasts were feeling empty due to losing volume after breastfeeding two children. I also felt my areolas were a little large anyway, and combined with the loss in volume, I just felt they looked hideous. It really affected my confidence. Wearing bikinis was a nightmare, and I was always covering up. I was so self-conscious, especially in the bedroom.

Aysha describes how her life changed after having breast enlargement and a lift.

Since having the surgery, my life now feels amazing. Physically my breasts are fuller and my areolas are smaller, but mentally I just feel much more confident in myself and in what I wear. I am able to travel and feel carefree about my breasts. I no longer feel the need to cover them up all the time. My confidence is the key thing that has changed for me. I am so much happier and feel like it has completely changed my life.

When asked what she would say to someone considering a breast enlargement and lift, Aysha was emphatic.

Just do it! If you are not feeling happy with how your breasts look, and they are genuinely making you feel down in the dumps, then just have them done. Personally, it was the best thing I have ever done. Before the surgery I found myself looking at my breasts and wishing for something better, but now I just don't have those worries anymore. The surgery is not as bad as people think. Just make sure you do your research and speak to your surgeon about all your questions and concerns. If you have low confidence, this will definitely give you the boost you need.

Breast Enhancement Procedures

Whether you want to enlarge your breasts, lift them, or reduce their size, here are the options to consider.

Breast Augmentation: Also known as augmentation mammoplasty, this can provide a beautiful, feminine silhouette and fullness of the breasts. The choices now available with the improved breast implants allow a plastic surgeon to enlarge and reshape small, disproportionate breasts, asymmetrical breasts, or misshapen breasts.

Women may select breast augmentation because of changes they experience in their breasts due to age, pregnancy, or weight loss. And by the way, certain surgeons offer a method to minimize your discomfort and get you back to your routine as quickly as a few days.

There are a number of options available to customize this procedure, which include rounded or teardrop implant shapes; multiple breast profiles; a silicone implant option; a saline implant option; "Gummy Bear" implants; and the location of the breast implant itself.

Your surgeon will examine the anatomy of the breast tissue, skin quality, and the extent of the desired enlargement in order to determine the appropriate incision location. He/she will also evaluate the amount and quality of glandular tissue and fat in the breasts to target the best location for them.

Breast Lift: Also referred to as mastopexy, a breast lift is a constellation procedure that provides women with choices to create their ideal breast shape and position. Often, undesirable changes in the breasts occur over time, causing them to lose volume, resulting in sagging.

The loss of volume can be due to pregnancy, breastfeeding, or weight change. This breast deflation is often accompanied by reduced elasticity in the breast tissue. All of these factors contribute to sagging of the breasts.

Your plastic surgeon will not only be lifting up the breast tissue and sculpting the breast mound, but will also modify the size of the areola, making it more proportionate and aesthetically pleasing.

 **Breast Reduction**: Also known as reduction mammaplasty surgery, this is a common procedure among women with enlarged breasts. Uniquely, it provides functional improvements and enhances the aesthetic appearance of the breasts. The goal of this procedure is to reduce the breasts so that they are proportionate to the rest of your body. Enlarged breasts can also cause many problems for women, including back, neck, and shoulder pain. Sometimes breasts are so large that they sag downwards, and in this case, a lift may be needed as well.

Fat Transfer (breast augmentation without implants): Patients who want to undergo a breast augmentation, or need to naturally restore contours, but want to avoid implants, may find that a fat transfer is a viable option. This procedure uses fat grafting techniques to transfer the fat from an area of your body that contains unwanted fat, such as your thighs, abdomen, or back and, after purification, injects the cleansed fat into the desired area. This is a more natural way to obtain acceptable results.

Implant Replacement

Women are discovering implants can be replaced to their advantage, particularly if dissatisfied with a former procedure.

Jennifer reveals:

> After my last child and breastfeeding for a year, my breasts looked
> "horrific" to me. There was a lot of loose skin, and I was so self-
> conscious about them. I work out, but my pecs were bothering
> me because the implant would rise up and the skin would sag
> off the implant. I could not have intercourse with my husband
> without it consuming me and would not get into certain positions
> because of it. I hated being naked around my husband. I work out
> and eat right, but this was the one thing I could not fix. I wanted
> to be confident in my body again. I wanted to be intimate with
> my husband and not worry about what my breasts were doing.

No longer being able to cope with these problems, Jennifer reached a
life-changing decision. "I decided to have my implants replaced and go
larger than previous, but still reasonable for my body." This time around,
she engaged in a good deal of research to find a plastic surgeon best
suited to her needs.

> I looked at reviews and pictures, as well as places they performed
> surgery and how long they had been in practice. This was my
> "baby" that I was going to be having, and I wanted to make sure
> she had the best.

> The plastic surgeon I ultimately chose took his time during
> the consultation to make sure he was able to answer all my
> questions and concerns. He had the best "bedside manner,"
> and in the before and after pictures I reviewed, his patients had
> that "natural" look.

Jennifer's surgery went smoothly, but she experienced some problems
during her recovery period.

> I did well with the pain and only took pain pills for the first two
> to three days, trying to sleep as much as I could. The worst part

for me was the stretching; it was very painful. I do have some slight numbness in areas from my armpit down to my elbows, but nothing that I notice daily.

Jennifer is quite pleased with how everything turned out.

I love my results! I am so happy with my surgery. I am more confident in myself. I know what is under my shirt (LOL), and that is all that matters. My husband obviously loves my breasts, but the confidence I have back in the bedroom, wearing lingerie and being naked again, makes it so worthwhile. We have that intimacy back that my head would not allow me to have.

She has words of advice for those considering breast augmentation.

I would tell anyone to do their research on plastic surgeons. You do not have to go to Beverly Hills to get the "best" doctor. Look at before and after pictures for the procedure you want done and read reviews.

I will probably have my breasts done one more time in another fifteen to twenty years, depending on how they look then. I may need a lift at that point after gravity has taken a toll on me (LOL). I am going to be forty-five in a few months, and I feel amazing.

Supersized to Natural

Breast enhancement procedures are more popular than ever. They remain one of the most sought-after cosmetic surgeries in many countries from the United States and Brazil to the UK and China. They're the subject of reality shows and tabloid spreads, and a recurrent topic of celebrity culture. But in terms of size, implants are actually getting smaller and appearing more "natural."

Studies also indicate that in the United States and the UK, demand for breast reduction procedures has grown—and according to Google Trends, the number of people searching for "breast reduction surgery" has been rising steadily in different countries since the onset of the pandemic in 2020.

The first breast enlargement surgery using silicone implants was performed in 1962, when **Timmie Jean Lindsey**, a thirty-year-old mother of six, was taken from a B cup to a C cup at Jefferson Davis Hospital in Houston, Texas. Lindsey had come into the hospital to have a tattoo removed from her breasts when doctors offered her the chance to get the first-of-its-kind procedure.

The times were ripe for a new kind of look. Barbie had hit the scene just a few years prior, and *Playboy* magazine was increasing in male and female readership. Throughout the 1950s, curvaceous Hollywood stars like Marilyn Monroe, Rita Hayworth, and Jayne Mansfield had America lusting after their hourglass figures and ample breasts, shaping ideals for feminine beauty.

By 2010, breast augmentation was the most popular form of plastic surgery in the United States. Over the years, many women also embraced implants as a tool to be noticed in an increasingly visual society. However, there's been a twist to the story in recent years, with unnaturally large fake breasts no longer a signifier of sexual liberation or individuality. They became synonymous with artificiality and tackiness. Most women don't want to be associated with that any longer.

The deflation of oversized breasts was also spurred by a shift in aesthetics. Simply, a new trend began taking hold—that of natural-looking breasts. The rise in popularity for a more athletic look—toned and slender— has perhaps further contributed to the demand for smaller breasts. This trend is largely borne out by celebrities who have opted for breast reductions. They include Drew Barrymore, Kris Jenner, Jennifer Connelly, Queen Latifah, and Patricia Heaton.

Patricia Heaton, the *Everybody Loves Raymond* star, had another reason for wanting breast reduction. She frankly said, "The fourth kid did me in. Some people are cool with the fact their bodies bear witness to this great thing they produce, their children, and I understand that. But on a personal level, it makes me feel better that my breasts are not down to my knees, especially when I'm undressed in front of my husband."

Can Breast Enhancement Change Your Life?

By her eighteenth birthday, **Laura** realized "the girls" weren't growing—but she pushed aside thoughts of breast implants. For eight years, she resisted the pressures of society, images of stars and starlets, and the focus on female anatomy. "It's everywhere in your face," said Laura (now much older). "I felt like less of a woman."

Laura finally did it—tossing the padded bras away forever and opting for silicone breast implants. "It may seem petty to some people, but felt I needed to do something about it," she related. "I didn't get a drastic implant, just one that suited me. I didn't want it to be, 'Look what she did.'"

When asked how she feels about her results, Laura enthusiastically responds. "I can't believe how real and how natural they look. I can't even describe how happy I am."

In fact, she adds that the preparation for breast-implant surgery pushed her into a healthier lifestyle. "I got into a vitamin regimen and quit smoking. It was a big opportunity for me to be a healthier person. It felt like everything was going in the right direction. It was so exciting."

What's Age Got to Do with It?

Wendi discusses the silicone implants she replaced with saline.

I am a sixty-two-year-old female and have come back to my surgeon for my second set of breast implants. My first set was done twenty-five years ago. They were silicone implants, and I was super happy with the results. After twenty-five years, they needed to be replaced, and this time I went with the saline implants. Once again, I couldn't be happier with the results. I definitely would recommend the saline implants over the silicone implants as I personally feel they are softer and are more natural looking."

Wendi raves about her plastic surgeon. "The patient care before and after the surgery was amazing, and I have had absolutely no problems since my surgery. Many thanks once again for the two wonderful experiences."

Breast Reconstruction

The goal of breast reconstruction is to restore one or both breasts to near normal shape, appearance, symmetry and size following mastectomy, lumpectomy or congenital deformities. Breast reconstruction generally falls into two categories: implant-based reconstruction or flap reconstruction. Implant reconstruction relies on breast implants to help form a new breast mound. Flap (or autologous) reconstruction uses the patient's own tissue from another part of the body to form a new breast.

"More than 70 percent of women who forgo reconstruction at the time of their breast surgery don't even know it's an option or may not have access to a plastic surgeon. These women are focused and worried about managing their diagnosis," says Gedge Rosson, director of breast reconstruction at Johns Hopkins.

Here are some important considerations that most people may not be aware of about **delayed breast reconstruction**:

- The vast majority of breast cancer survivors are good candidates.

- **Breast reconstruction can improve your quality of life.** Some patients don't have the opportunity or are not interested in reconstruction when they are first treated for breast cancer. However, breast reconstruction is available at any point, and it often helps patients feel better about their overall experiences, as well as what their bodies have had to face. Leading studies that compared quality-of-life assessments for women before and after breast reconstruction reveal that reconstruction, whether immediate or delayed, can greatly improve a woman's sense of wholeness and well-being.

- **Prostheses can be cumbersome**. Patients that opt for prostheses often find that they're heavy and hard to fit with their clothing. Prostheses may also require regular replacement. Breast reconstruction can be a permanent solution for restoring your breasts to a more natural shape and size. Breast reconstruction can also alleviate pain and chest tightness associated with radiation treatment and, in some cases, actually improve nipple sensation.

- **You don't have to live with jagged, indented scars**. Innovations in breast reconstruction surgery over the last decade have greatly improved appearance, including reducing the number of indentations and appearance of scars.

- **It's okay to wait**. In many cases, your reconstructed breasts will look just as good whether you had reconstruction during your mastectomy or after. Even if you were counseled against breast reconstruction at the time of your treatment, advances in reconstructive techniques may qualify you for the procedure.

- **You can pick an option that fits your lifestyle**. Your surgeon can work with you to create a customized treatment plan to suit your preferences. For example, you can choose between having breast reconstruction in one longer surgery or several shorter and less invasive ones. You'll also have the choice to enable your breasts to be reconstructed using your own tissue from the belly, thighs, buttocks, or back. Additionally, you can select reconstruction using implants made of saline or silicone.

- **It's covered by insurance**. Health care costs are often a primary concern for patients facing any surgical procedure. For breast reconstruction after breast cancer, it doesn't have to be. Federal law requires that breast reconstruction, in addition to other post-mastectomy benefits, be covered by medical insurance.

Louise's Story

"Dance is one of those things that it doesn't matter how good you are," said **Louise**. "You never stop learning. There's always more. This is what I love to do. I want to enjoy the use of this body until I can't use this body any longer, so that's what pushes me."

Louise was diagnosed with invasive tubulolobular carcinoma after a routine mammogram. She had a double mastectomy followed by reconstruction with expanders placed for implants. After that, Louise had chemotherapy because her doctors found a positive lymph node following surgery. Ten days after her first chemo appointment, Louise became septic, and one of the expanders was infected. (*How much must this woman have endured?*) At that point, she was referred to a plastic surgeon who informed her about natural tissue breast reconstruction.

> I'm very fortunate. I have a wonderful marriage and two children and six grandchildren. But I'm also a very high-energy person, and dance is my happy place. I underwent the DIEP flap surgery, and it was the smartest thing I ever did. When I finished the chemo, I was told that implants were no longer an option for me. Fortunately, I found one of the few surgeons who was doing DIEP flap reconstruction on very thin women.

When asked about her experience with the DIEP flap surgery and recovery, she provided an honest assessment.

The first two weeks are hard. But by the third week, you're able to function on your own. Yes, it hurts. There are surgical drains. There is the surgical bra. There are compression garments. There's all that stuff to deal with, but you can handle it. By the third week, it's much better, and then every week is a huge difference. You wake up on week four, and you feel so much better.

Louise explains how she has fared after natural breast tissue reconstruction.

It's a big surgery, but within six weeks, I was dancing again. Maybe I wasn't dancing full speed, but I was dancing and moving, and I've never had a problem with movement of my arms or using my abdominal muscles. I'm very pleased that's the route that I ended up choosing. Most important, I know I will never have surgery ever again. This is it. And what's amazing to me is that I think my figure is far better now than it was before I ever had cancer.

Dr. Hardesty: Breasts "sag" or "hang" because the "skin bra" is larger than the breast tissue. Over time, the weight of breast tissue can continue to stretch the skin and acts like a "rock in a sock." Some women develop breasts that sag, but more often, the cycle of expansion and contraction of breast tissue (during pregnancy and/or after weight loss) results in a permanent stretching of the skin. The once full and rounded breast can take the shape of a bowling pin. Technically, the "viscoelastic" properties of the skin have been irreversibly altered. A mastopexy, or breast lift, involves shaping the breast, repositioning the nipple areolar complex (NAC), and when needed, reducing the NAC size. It also removes excess skin that causes the sag of the breast. The nipple is left connected to the breast tissue.

Depending on your interests, the shape and the look of the breasts, your chosen plastic surgeon will decide what type of mastopexy is required. It is common for plastic surgeons to request model photos to better understand a patient's desires.

Dr. Polakof: Breast enhancement can play a major role in how a woman perceives herself. It truly is an extension of inner beauty and self-confidence. Having said this, there are perils, which usually stem from practice marketing, lower pricing, and doctors who promote unrealistic expectations. When it comes to breast surgery, it is more important than ever to actually speak with a surgeon's patients to gain their perspective.

CHAPTER 17

NONSURGICAL BODY PROCEDURES AND ATTAINING BEAUTIFUL SKIN

"My transformation represents more than what is just skin deep;
it represents my motivation, drive, and willingness
to constantly improve."

—Jinder Mahal

It's comforting to know that in plastic surgery, one can choose an alternative without necessarily sacrificing quality. Of course, obtaining the desired result may be deemed necessary as a surgical procedure, but when it comes to body contouring and other less invasive treatments, there are viable options and perhaps even more suitable choices.

With the newest contouring technologies, plastic surgeons can help their patients reduce cellulite and fat and give them an enhanced figure. The first option we will examine is a treatment known as **UltraShape® Power**.

UltraShape® Power is an FDA-cleared treatment for noninvasive reduction in stomach circumference and fat reduction in the abdomen, flanks, and thighs. It gently destroys fat by delivering non-thermal ultrasound energy waves that are:

- **Focused**—delivering ultrasound energy to tissue within a precise focal volume at a controlled depth (no needles, surgery, or diet necessary)

- **Pulsed**—mechanical non-thermal effect resulting in minimal elevation of treated tissue for a truly comfortable and gentle treatment experience

- **Selective**—precisely targeting fat cells while blood vessels, nerves, and surrounding tissue remain largely unaffected

Since UltraShape® Power selectively and precisely targets fat cells, blood vessels, nerves, and surrounding tissue is largely unharmed. There are no reported cases of lumping, shelving, or other contouring deformities. It's actually a walk-in, walk-out procedure which is virtually painless. In a recent clinical study, the average reported pain level was 1 on a 10-point scale. Thousands of plastic surgery patients have experienced benefits from this treatment and are often able to eliminate extra body fat that even diets and gym exercises can't shed.

Full results will be achieved after going through a series of three to four treatments. But does it provide the dramatic results of liposuction? Likely not; however, many patients with lesser challenges are quite pleased.

A second option to consider is **VelaShape® III,** which is a noninvasive radio frequency (RF) treatment with suction that is pain-free and requires no downtime. With over ten years of clinical experience, more than five million independent treatments, and the most published studies of any medical body-shaping device, VelaShape is one of the most recognized noninvasive body-shaping treatments on the market today.

The VelaShape® III procedure is comfortable, comparable to a hot stone massage, and the treatment requires less than one hour. It's geared to reduce or eliminate cellulite, loose skin after liposuction, and wrinkles. This treatment can be effectively utilized on areas like abdomen, thighs, buttocks, neck, and arms.

Many patients can start to see almost immediate promise, but it often takes several treatments for optimal results to be seen. Occasional maintenance treatments are required to maintain or enhance the initial results.

Another consideration in the VelaShape class is **ThermiTight®**, used to shrink skin and connective tissue in a predictable manner. It uses the science of heat to transform tissue in desirable ways to provide a leaner look, a tighter jawline and neck, and sleeker arms, thighs, and abdomens.

Surgeons who utilize fillers and toxins to reshape the aging face can now use ThermiTight to inject heat in a similar way, reducing sagging skin laxity throughout the body. Each patient is unique, thus there is a range of healing responses. The numbing fluid will need to be absorbed by the body over the first day or two, so patients might look a bit swollen. The puncture sites will heal without scarring as any small wound would.

The treated area will be wrapped to keep it under light compression for twenty-four hours, perhaps longer if your surgeon feels you need it. You may be sensitive to heat in the treated area for a few days. Additionally, there is sometimes tenderness lasting a few weeks and a firmness, called induration, that will fade with time. Often, this indicates an excellent response.

Many patients return to daily activities immediately since there is little to no downtime associated with this procedure. Most recipients of ThermiTight begin to notice improvements within the first week of treatment, but the optimal results will be seen within a couple months.

CoolSculpting and EMSCULPT are two additional nonsurgical body procedures that have risen in popularity. CoolSculpting's primary goal is to reduce fat, whereas EMSCULPT tones muscle.

CoolSculpting uses controlled cooling to "freeze" targeted fat cells in the treatment area, which are then metabolized by the body. The process is called cryolipolysis and often works because fat cells begin dying when cooled to lower temperatures. There is minimal downtime following the treatment, and few side effects are reported, such as redness and swelling.

An EMSCULPT treatment, on the other hand, uses advanced, high-intensity focused electromagnetic technology to stimulate thousands of involuntary muscle contractions during a single treatment session.

It claims to compare to completing twenty thousand sit-ups in thirty minutes, toning the abdominal and gluteus muscles. (This claim is appealing, but subject to question.) After the treatment, you can expect to feel soreness similar to what you might experience after an extremely strenuous workout. The procedure does burn fat, since EMSCULPT is primarily for muscle toning. Improvements may reveal themselves after about two months.

Cautionary Tale: Supermodel Linda Evangelista

Although body contouring procedures are known to benefit some patients, there are many less skilled, inexperienced doctors who offer these procedures—and there are risks involved. You really must discuss what is most appropriate for your body with a board-certified plastic surgeon.

A good case in point is Linda Evangelista, a supermodel who became famous in the 1990s. She claims to be "brutally disfigured" and "unrecognizable" after a CoolSculpting procedure turned her into a recluse.

In an Instagram post, she referred to filing a lawsuit, saying that she was taking "a big step toward righting a wrong that I have suffered and have kept to myself for over five years." She added, "To my followers who have wondered why I have not been working while my peers' careers have been thriving, the reason is that I was brutally disfigured by Zeltiq's CoolSculpting procedure, which did the opposite of what it promised."

Ms. Evangelista said that, after the fat-freezing procedure, she developed paradoxical adipose hyperplasia, a side effect in which patients experience firm tissue masses in the treatment areas. She claimed the cosmetic procedure left her "permanently deformed even after undergoing two painful, unsuccessful corrective surgeries." She said she had not been told of the risk.

"PAH has not only destroyed my livelihood; it has sent me into a cycle of deep depression, profound sadness, and the lowest depths of self-loathing," she reported. "In the process, I have become a recluse."

In all fairness, there have been positive patient testimonials about the benefits of CoolSculpting—but Linda's case is a good example of the importance of discussing your desires with a plastic surgeon, who usually better understands body anatomy with respect to aesthetics and which option will best suit your needs.

Despite all the leaps in technology, fat-reduction procedures are not magic, fat-zapping unicorns. They are intended as a refinement for people within ten pounds of their goal weight, not as a weight-loss method. Liposuction still reigns supreme when it comes to medical intervention for fat elimination. With body procedures, the biggest source of disappointment is that the nonsurgical treatment often didn't do as much as hoped.

Laser Hair Removal

If you're not happy with shaving, tweezing, or waxing to remove unwanted hair, laser hair removal may be an option worth considering.

Laser hair removal is one of the most commonly performed cosmetic procedures in the US. It beams highly concentrated light into hair follicles. The pigment in the follicles absorb the light, which destroys the unwanted hair.

GentleLase Pro is a procedure that addresses all of your hair removal needs. It employs a flash lamp technology which stimulates an alexandrite crystal to create a wavelength of light. This wavelength is delivered to the patient's skin, along with a burst of cryogen that cools the epidermal layer of skin to a comfortable level. This allows for fast and effective treatment.

The 755nm alexandrite laser targets the melanin (dark pigment) in the hair, effectively destroying the hair follicle at the root and preventing future hair growth. Since hair grows in cycles, a series of three to four sessions about four to six weeks apart is recommended because hair grows in three stages. Thus, hair needs to be in the "growth" stage in order for the hairs on your body to be ablated and carried out for optimal permanent hair removal. In addition to removing hair from the body (including beard hair), this versatile laser can also treat leg veins, pigmented lesions, and spider and facial veins. Patients will see some parafollicular edema and feel perhaps like they were in the sun. This is why a cool compress or gel pack may be applied. Any redness or swelling should resolve in a few hours.

Motif Laser: Powered by the proprietary elōs technology, Motif is the only mechanization using combined energies of radio frequency (RF) and electrical energy to gently remove hair from all lighter hair tones. Since the Motif is "color blind," it can treat darker skin colors and tones without damaging them.

The hair follicles are precisely targeted and destroyed using the revolutionary elōs combination of bi-polar radio frequency with an 810-diode laser. Motif LHR selectively targets the hair follicle while protecting the surrounding tissue, so it's safe and effective for all skin colors, tones, and types. Hair growth is reduced after each treatment. The number of treatments required will vary, depending on the location and size of the area being treated as well as the individual rate at which your hair grows. This is due to the fact that hair grows in three stages and needs to be in the "growth" stage in order for the Motif treatment to be successful. The hairs on your body are not always at the same stage, so you'll need to undergo a few treatments, an average of four to six weeks apart, to catch all of the light-colored hairs in their growth stage. The treatment is known to be safe, without any downtime.

Attaining Beautiful Skin

When it comes to skin care goals, the word "glowing" seems to universally rank first. There are natural ways to attain and preserve beautiful, glowing skin, but often you need a little help from your friends (aestheticians and skin care specialists employed by plastic surgery practices).

Natural Methods

Use a safe, mineral-based sunscreen daily.

Light exfoliation—removing the outer layer of excess dead skin cells will help smooth skin texture.

Protect your gut. Anything that's not healthy for your gut (i.e., sugar and processed food) can lead to gut microbial imbalance, triggering oxidative stress and inflammatory processes. These imbalances also manifest as skin issues.

Incorporate healthy fats into your diet. Those found in nuts, flaxseed, and avocados can help to create healthy, strong cell membranes. Eat antioxidant-rich foods such as leafy greens and berries.

Apply moisturizers right after bathing on your face and body to seal in moisture and prevent dry skin.

One of the best topical ingredients for glowing skin is vitamin C, which works on all skin types to even out and brighten tone.

Stay hydrated. Drinking enough water is essential for skin health.

Get your beauty sleep. Research has shown that poor sleep quality can contribute to increased signs of skin aging (fine lines and wrinkles).

As helpful as these natural methods can be, many of us simply need a little help from our friends from time to time to create and maintain beautiful, glowing skin. The majority of plastic surgery practices feature licensed aestheticians, or highly skilled skin care specialists, who are under the supervision and guidance of a board-certified plastic surgeon. Here are important skin rejuvenation options available through these practices.

Topical Skin Rejuvenation Medications

Tretinoin (Retin-A® and Renova®). Medical-grade Tretinoin requires a prescription, but Tretinoin has a long track record of being cost-efficient, effective, and a reliable method for increasing skin collagen production, resulting in a more youthful skin look.

Hydroquinone has a history of success for lightening pigment irregularities often referred to as sun, liver, and age spots (or freckles). It works by decreasing the amount of melanin produced by melanocytes, which determines your skin tone. In situations of hyperpigmentation, more melanin is present. By reducing melanin production, your skin will potentially become more evenly toned over time.

Topical highly concentrated **vitamin C serum** is proven to boost radiance and neutralize free radicals that lead to skin aging. Vitamin C serum is specially formulated and packaged to have maximal effect when applied on the skin.

Medically Supervised Facials

Thanks to increased consumer awareness, many women are turning to medical facials over those traditional beauty facials found in spas or salons. Medical facials incorporate mild peeling agents, advanced equipment to hydrate and exfoliate the skin, and specific techniques such as radiofrequency current to firm up skin.

Before suggesting treatment, the plastic surgeon and/or medical aesthetician first analyzes your skin and then makes a tailored recommendation. The amalgamation of products and machines, including intense pulsed light (IPL), ensures that the treatment permeates deeper epidermal layers and targets the dermal layer of the skin.

Microdermabrasion

Microdermabrasion is a procedure used to treat acne scars, skin discoloration, sun damage, and stretch marks by removing the top layer of skin. Microdermabrasion benefits include improvement in the skin's texture and appearance. A microdermabrasion treatment is typically performed by a plastic surgeon's aesthetician using a handheld device that gently removes the top layer of skin. Because it deeply exfoliates, microdermabrasion can improve the tone and texture of your skin.

If a series of treatments is performed (which is usually recommended), you should notice your skin tone smoothing out and may see a softening of fine lines and superficial wrinkles. Microdermabrasion can also help fight sun damage and enable anti-aging creams to be more effective.

Chemical Peels

Like microdermabrasion, chemical peels address a variety of topical skin issues. What differs between the two is how the outer layer of the skin is removed to find the new skin underneath. While microdermabrasion gently removes the epidermis by suction, chemical peels use a chemical solution to dissolve the skin off.

Chemical peels treat a diversity of conditions, including acne, fine lines, crow's feet, brown spots, sagging skin, wrinkles, blemishes, hyperpigmentation, and melasma. A chemical peel works at a deeper level than microdermabrasion, revealing newer skin underneath. Because of this, it does require a few days of peeling.

The choice between these two treatments depends on what you expect to achieve. If you want an affordable and fast option, microdermabrasion is typically a better selection. But if you prefer something that lasts longer, a chemical peel might better suit your needs.

We earlier discussed the benefits of injectables, fillers, and lasers in our nonsurgical facial rejuvenation chapter, and these modalities should be taken into consideration for skin revitalization as well. However, the bottom line is to select a plastic surgery practice which specializes in all these procedures, rather than another medical branch which may be limited in its capabilities.

Celebrity Go-to Skin Beauty Treatments

The various celebrity beauty treatments are as different as the A-listers who love them, but every therapy strives more or less toward the same goal: glowing skin. Often working with unconventional methods, these treatments themselves are a fascinating look into a sect of the beauty industry often obscured from public view.

Meghan Markle: There's a lot to admire about Meghan Markle and the perennial glow she exhibits. But her sharp jawline and taut skin might be more accessible than you'd think. Before her marriage to Prince Harry, Meghan was very vocal about her love for the **buccal massage**, a mouth muscle massage. Buccal fat pads, located just below your cheekbones, contribute to that full-faced, baby-like look typically associated with youth. A beauty professional massages that area of the face, both outside and inside the mouth, to stimulate blood flow, drain any excess fluid, and encourage collagen production. The end result is a sharp-looking jawline worthy of its own crown.

Kim Kardashian: The **vampire facial**, designed to utilize the client's own blood as a key component of the process, became a beauty and pop culture standard the moment Kim Kardashian uploaded a photo of herself undergoing the treatment, seemingly covered in blood. In reality, it's a Dermapen packed with nano-sized needles to grab a person's own platelet-packed plasma, which helps stimulate collagen and improve skin elasticity. Kim did, however, reveal that she "regrets" the facial because of the pain factor.

Rihanna: Have you ever seen Rihanna when she doesn't emit a glow on the red carpet? Of course not, and it's largely thanks to this eight-hundred-dollar facial she swears by before big events. But because this is Rihanna we're talking about, it's no ordinary facial. The treatment is known as the **electro-fusion facial** and combines a series of proprietary micro-current, light, and radiofrequency treatments to sculpt the face and coax out an otherworldly radiance.

Gwyneth Paltrow: Known as the queen of "Goop," Gwyneth has tried quite a few homeopathic and obscure remedies over the years, but her **bee sting therapy** might take the cake. As the name would suggest, she subjected herself to actual bee stings in an effort to reduce inflammation. "I've been stung by bees. It's a thousands-of-years-old treatment called **apitherapy**," Gwyneth claims. "People use it to get rid of inflammation and scarring. It's actually pretty incredible if you research it. But, man, it's painful." With the very real risk of life-threatening allergic reactions, this treatment is not worth serious consideration.

Beyoncé: Her skin is always glowing and immaculate, which she attributes to **hydrafacials**, which combine salicylic, glycolic, and hyaluronic acids to eat away at dead skin, bacteria, and debris with the help of a suction vacuum. Her aesthetician also alternates a rush of oxygen and antioxidants to ensure nothing about the treatment is too irritating. However, unless you have a celebrity-size treasure chest and an entourage of beauty specialists to draw from, your most cost-effective and dependable option is to visit a local plastic surgery office to gain knowledgeable advice about which treatments are most suitable for you.

Dr. Hardesty: We are all born with a certain number of fat cells. As we gain weight, they increase in size, and conversely, when we lose weight, the fat cells shrink. The difference between weight loss and fat reduction is that weight loss doesn't reduce the number of fat cells, while fat reduction does. In essence, fat reduction ensures that the fat cells that might gain weight are eliminated for good, regardless of your weight, and thus, your body shape will permanently remain thinner.

In terms of a nonsurgical fat-reduction treatment, I do favor UltraShape as an excellent option. These treatments are performed on a "walk-in, walk-out" basis with absolutely no downtime and no pain. It's also the highest rated nonsurgical fat-reduction technology in the US.

Dr. Polakof: So many women are paying exorbitant prices for department store and over-the-counter beauty products to enhance their skin. The problem is that most of these lotions and creams fall short of expectations promoted by salespeople.

The same is true of so-called "medical-grade" skin care. Though many of them are supported by clinical studies, medical-grade products can only use ingredients approved for over-the-counter use.

Prescription skincare products have been approved by the FDA and can only be prescribed by a licensed physician. These products have rigorous scientific backing, proving their safety and efficacy for treating medical skin conditions. You will likely end up spending about the same for prescribed products compared to those which are less effective for your skin.

CHAPTER 18

PLASTIC SURGERY FOR MEN

"There is nothing noble in being superior to your fellow man; true nobility is being superior to your former self."
—Ernest Hemingway

Okay, fellows, we know you probably don't stand in the locker room and chat with your buddies about your double chin or love handles. But if you're being honest, it's not uncommon for insecurities to arise for men, just like they do for the ladies. While women tend to talk more openly about their facial and body concerns, there appears to be a growing number of men who are also interested in enabling their inner beauty to rise to the surface.

According to the American Society of Plastic Surgeons, cosmetic and plastic surgery procedures performed on men have increased by 28 percent since 2000. Even though men may not openly discuss aesthetic procedures, it's obvious that plastic surgery has become increasingly of interest. Though there are a variety of surgical procedures they are turning to, the four top plastic surgery categories for men are facial surgeries, male breast reduction, liposuction, and hair restoration.

Facial Improvements for Men

Men care about their appearance more than ever and focus on putting their best face forward. To do so, many are turning to surgical procedures to help achieve the appearance they want. Some choose to fix certain bothersome features, like their noses, whether they were born with one that is not personally appealing or need help repairing it after an injury.

Rhinoplasty, often referred to as a "nose job," is a surgical procedure that aesthetically reshapes the nose and has been one of the most popular plastic surgeries among men for some time.

Men who wish to recapture a more youthful facial appearance may turn to an eyelid lift (blepharoplasty) to remove or reposition the skin around the eye. Or they may kick it up a notch and undergo a full facelift, technically known as a rhytidectomy. This procedure lifts sagging skin, tightens facial muscles, and reduces the effects of time and gravity, often taking years off the face.

These three facial procedures are covered thoroughly in our chapter entitled "Facial Rejuvenation: Achieving a 'Natural Look.'"

Male Breast Reduction

 Let's be honest: Every man secretly wants to look like Tarzan or "The Rock" (Dwayne Johnson). And most men don't want their chest to jiggle or droop or appear like a feminine breast. However, "man boobs," a condition medically referred to as gynecomastia, affects an estimated 40 to 60 percent of men.

Some fellows could spend every waking minute in the gym and still struggle to get that coveted, rock-hard chest. Because of this, more men are undergoing male breast reduction surgery.

Gynecomastia surgery is the procedure to help reduce the excess tissue found in the abnormally large male breast. The choice of the technique is heavily dependent on the possibility of later skin redundancy.

Liposuction Technique: This procedure is best used if the gynecomastia is primarily caused by excess fatty tissue. It is performed by making small incisions around the area, inserting a small surgical tool, and loosening the fat cells to vacuum them out.

Excision Technique: This approach is advantageous when the excess skin and glandular breast tissue need to be removed.

Combination: In certain cases, both techniques are required to effectively remedy gynecomastia.

Recovery from male breast reduction is rather quick. Most men return to work in the next day or so. A small compression garment, the size of an undershirt, is worn for six weeks, and the patient is able to return to normal activities without limitations.

How I Got Rid of My Boobs After Nine Years of Struggle

Oskar is a personal trainer, but he didn't always have a "ripped" body. He recalls:

> It's difficult to feel comfortable in your own skin when you constantly have to hide your chest. It's even more difficult to feel happy when you avoid getting intimate with others because

of your soft chest. I know because I used to have man boobs throughout all my teenage years into adulthood.

Oskar explains that gynecomastia can be severe as the gland pushes out your nipples. "The puffy nipples are especially visible when you are wearing a tight T-shirt, sit down, or when you are in humid and hot weather."

He combatted his condition with hormone therapy, which still left him with moderate gynecomastia. Thus, it was time for surgery, but he was wise in doing a good deal of research. "Gynecomastia surgery is not just something you do. It's something that needs to be done right. You don't want to mess up your chest for life because you didn't do your research. There are plenty of horror stories out there of guys who had horrible results."

Oskar chose a board-certified plastic surgeon with extensive gynecomastia surgery experience. "Today, they are *gone*, and for the first time in nine years, my chest looks exactly the way I always wanted it to."

Ralph has a similar story.

> I was always uncomfortable with my chest, but I thought that I was chubby and had "man boobs" from just fat. I've always had "pointy nipples" where the areola grows in size and sticks out more when it is warm than when cold. I was definitely ridiculed for it when younger (like at the pool or when wearing tighter shirts), and even as I became older, I noticed people staring at my chest in the gym or at the beach. I thought that the problem would go away when I got into shape. After all, I thought that it was just fat tissue. However, over the course of gaining muscle and losing weight, I noticed that the "boobs" became more visible and did not reduce in size much when I lost weight.

Ralph did his research and finally decided to have gynecomastia surgery.

It was my first time under general anesthesia, so I was a bit anxious about it, but the doctors and nurses were excellent and made me feel very comfortable. The surgery was over in an hour, and I don't remember a thing. I was awake and out the door after thirty to forty-five minutes of recovery from the anesthesia. They gave me diazepam and hydrocodone to reduce the pain and help me relax and sleep while I recovered.

Is he pleased? "I am very happy with my results. I would really encourage any guy dealing with gynecomastia issues to go see a top-notch doctor like I did."

Save that Spare Tire for the Car

Some men may call it their spare tire or may refer to the condition as "love handles" or the dreaded "beer belly." Whatever the description, it's not something most men are particularly fond of. Perhaps you have always been a fairly fit fellow, but as aging occurs, you can't seem to get rid of that extra bulge. Or you might work out like a Tasmanian devil, yet those trouble spots refuse to go away. Interestingly, that "spare tire" can actually be due to hormonal changes which can cause this area to become very dense and resistant to diet and exercise.

Liposuction is usually the procedure of choice for this condition. You may recall from our chapter entitled "Body Contouring" that liposuction is performed through small, inconspicuous incisions. First, diluted local anesthesia is infused to reduce bleeding and trauma. Then a thin hollow tube, or cannula, is inserted through the incisions to loosen excess fat using a controlled back and forth motion and sucking it out.

The procedure itself can be performed efficiently and effectively and is fairly painless after the tumescent fluid has been injected. Typically, men return to daily activities and non-strenuous work within a few days following the procedure and wear a compression garment for a minimum of six weeks. Results are often seen immediately but may take a few months to appreciate the final outcome as the skin contours to the new shape.

Matt's Liposuction—His First Surgery

Matt is from Long Island and lost fifty pounds by following a strict diet and exercise regimen. He states, "I had worked so hard on my body to get myself to a place where I liked what I saw in the mirror, but there was this one area of stubborn fat that I just couldn't get rid of, so my surgeon suggested liposuction."

Matt reveals it was his first time.

It was actually the first surgery I've ever had, so I had no clue what to expect, but it was very straightforward, and I felt very safe throughout. I had my procedure under general anesthesia, and when I woke up, I was actually comfortable. I had very little discomfort during the entire recovery process. I'd booked a week out of work to give myself time to recuperate, but I actually didn't even need that long. I had time to relax and get a few chores done before I went back to the office, which was excellent!

He is apparently quite satisfied.

I'm really happy with how it's turned out. I think it's one of those things that you notice so much more on yourself than on anyone else. When I look back at the photos of myself before I had the surgery and compare them to how I look now, I can see a massive difference. Not only in how the area looks, but also in my attitude. It's a small procedure that's made a big difference in my confidence.

How Hair Loss in Men Affects Self-Esteem

There are many reasons for hair loss in men. Alopecia can occur due to hormonal problems, mechanical follicle damage, autoimmune conditions, or as a result of chemotherapy. The most common cause of male hair loss is androgenic alopecia (also known as male pattern baldness). In this condition, the scalp becomes more sensitive to the hormone dihydrotestosterone (DHT), which shortens hair growth cycle length and reduces hair follicle output. The result is fewer hairs growing over time in certain areas, like on the top of the head and over the temples. The hairs that do grow are thinner and more breakable than before.

According to the US National Library of Medicine, approximately 50 percent of Caucasian men experience male pattern baldness. The condition runs in families and is more likely to happen as you get older.

Hair loss has been affecting men's self-esteem for centuries, if not longer. In ancient times, long, thick hair was a symbol of masculinity and vitality, so it makes sense that men are psychologically affected by hair loss today, particularly with social media and the emphasis upon a virile male appearance. Additionally, hair loss symbolizes aging and debility, which is why psychologists believe that men start feeling more depressed as their hair starts falling out. Multiple studies have linked male pattern hair loss to lowered self-esteem and decreased confidence. A study in the *International Journal of Trichology* found that androgenic alopecia lowered the quality of life for many men, with particular effects in the areas of self-perception and interpersonal relations. In fact, hair loss in men can affect self-esteem to the extent that a man believes his appearance to be an important part of what makes him a worthwhile or valuable person. Fortunately, significant advances in the field of transplantation have been made recently which enable men to have hair with a natural appearance.

Male Hair Restoration

The global hair restoration industry is expected to reach $32.4 billion by 2026, growing at a compounded rate of 22.7 percent annually. Incredibly, every thirteenth man will opt for hair transplant surgery in his lifetime.

Although hair loss can be caused by a number of factors, thinning hair is particularly bothersome to men because of our culture's fixation on youth. As a result, many men who face hair loss feel pressured to do something about their condition before it becomes a bigger, more noticeable issue. With some men, it's also a matter of personal self-esteem when what they see in the mirror does not match the internal representation of themselves. Women may term this "inner beauty," but with men, it's "inner pride."

One of the most effective male restoration procedures is called "Advanced FUE Hair Transplantation." FUE procedures utilize hair follicles removed one by one from the donor and placed in the recipient area (top of scalp, hairline, crown). Follicles taken from the donor area (back of the scalp) are genetically immune to the effects of DHT (dihydrotestosterone, the hormone linked to hair loss) and retain this genetic attribute even after being transplanted to the recipient areas.

The difference is not in the area of hair growth, but how the donor area is harvested, either as a strip of the scalp or by small, individual graft extractions. Using the FUE technique leaves no linear scar. Overall, patient reviews have been impressive. In particular, patients are surprisingly pleased with the speed and efficiency of the FUE systems.

In addition to no visible scaring or stitches, the FUE results appear natural and seem to be permanent. The procedure is minimally invasive, with no downtime and fast recovery. Many plastic surgery practices now offer advanced FUE.

Brian's Crowning Achievement

Brian explains his motivation to seek hair restoration.

I started losing my hair—in the crown—when I was in my early fifties. At some point, it became a large area of no hair at all, and I didn't like the way I looked. I envied men with full heads of hair keeping them still looking young. The hair on the front appeared fine. So I decided to go through the procedure. Immediately following my hair procedure, I had *no* pain! Some minor blood spotting on my pillow, which I remedied by using a plastic trash liner over my pillow. My actual recovery time was about a week.

Brian is pleased with his results. "The hair on my crown is now about two-thirds full, which is a terrific improvement. If I was younger and single, I might opt for another round to fill it in, but I'm happy with the way it looks presently. And it's all *my* hair! I feel more confident because I feel good about how I look."

Steve is another hair transplant patient who shares Brian's views. "I really didn't want to lose my hair and become bald like my father. The result of hair restoration was excellent. My confidence level is much greater—and I am often told I look younger than my age."

Inner Beauty: Male and Female Comparisons

Inner beauty is important overall—but the definition of inner beauty also depends on your gender. In order to be considered attractive, men are expected to have the following traits: intelligent, knowledgeable, wise, funny, entertaining, and happy.

The shocking fact is that, through the eyes of both genders, at every age, women's top personality traits remain fairly consistent (and are more about what they do for others than who they actually are): caring, compassionate, generous, sincere, trusting, and altruistic.

The idea of beauty is always shifting. Mainstream television, media outlets, and social media have had us believing for years that only a select few are blessed with the gift of beauty and that their depiction of beauty is something we should aspire to. Look at the influencer culture and how it perpetuates unrealistic images.

However, more recent studies reveal that both men and women are now placing more value on what's on the inside. Be that as it may, despite gender and age, both men and women continue to believe outward appearance fuels success. At the same time, many people still feel expectations of beauty are unrealistic. This perception is significantly greater for women, in general, but resides mostly among older generations. A fascinating point to be made, though, is that younger people feel those expectations are almost as unrealistic for men as women. Is this a function of their age and lack of "real-life" experiences, or is the tide changing? Unsurprisingly, perhaps, gender also plays a role in shaping beauty perceptions. Men put a bit more importance on looks, though "who people are on the inside" is still the primary influence.

Dr. Hardesty: With respect to male insecurity attributed to hair loss, the modern technology of FUE is a relatively new but proven automated follicular unit extraction (FUE) and hair transplant system. With greater precision, it has markedly improved the harvesting of hair follicles without having to incur a large incision from ear to ear, with no need for sutures/staples (or their removal), while reducing complications and decreasing recovery time. Using the advanced follicular unit extraction (FUE) hair transplant technology has also dramatically improved accuracy and speed over the previously used manual extraction and non-sophisticated instrumentation. This results in a more robust hair graft which can be implanted sooner. It's a permanent solution, thus over time, a man's own hair will continue to grow naturally and continue to blend.

Dr. Polakof: My research indicates that, by and large, a man's concept of inner beauty is slowly beginning to evolve. Many men believe that beauty consists in strength of character. You are beautiful in the truest sense of the word if you help those who are going through hardships in life. If you respect others, irrespective of their wealth or poverty, and if you talk politely to people, you then deserve to be recognized for your inner beauty.

Thus, more men are shifting their perspective to embody the concept that beauty consists in goodness of character. It lies in the strength of inner character. It has less to do with exterior appearance. A person who is not physically appealing can be beautiful if he or she has a "heart of gold."

"It is not the beauty of a building you should look at, it's the construction of the foundation that will stand the test of time."
—David Allan Coe

CHAPTER 19

PLASTIC SURGERY FOR TEENS

"It takes courage to grow up and become who you really are."
—e. e. cummings

Bombarded by media images of perfect bodies, from Botox to breast implants, teenagers as young as thirteen are turning to plastic surgery to get bigger lips, smaller noses, lifted breasts, and other procedures. In fact, young people have become so open about their choice to undergo such elective procedures that some have posted video of themselves going under the knife on their social media accounts. One teenage girl even went on Snapchat and filmed herself live getting a liposuction procedure.

"I think we live in the generation where we equate our self-worth and value with literally every numerical value that's on a page," one young woman said during an interview. "So yeah, we see who's getting likes, who's getting followers, and we assume that that's the right path."

Ryan was fifteen when he got his ears surgically pinned back in an otoplasty procedure he said changed his life, giving him new confidence after years of being bullied for having big ears. "In the past, I didn't have the courage to stand up for myself," he said. "But after the surgery, I won't let anyone mess with me."

Ella, nineteen, was so excited about the idea of getting her lips done that she filmed it for her YouTube channel, where she told her viewers afterward: "I love them so much! Very good experience overall. Highly recommend."

However, Ella later admitted, "I definitely do think that I kind of fell victim to these beauty standards perpetuated by pop culture and social media. It's hard to think about the fact that I had to do this to feel this way about myself."

But for every surgical success, medical experts warn there are nightmare scenarios. Some of these are serious, causing infections and other complications.

Teenage Body Dysmorphia

A small subset of teens develop a preoccupation with looks that goes beyond basic anxiety. For these teens, one aspect of their bodies becomes so disturbing and overwhelming that it dominates the focus of their existence. If this behavior persists for a long period of time, they may be suffering from teenage body-dysmorphic disorder, a mental health issue that can grow stronger with time and cause severe damage.

Teenage body-dysmorphic disorder has also been closely linked to suicide. The young person grows more convinced that her or his body parts are hideous and unavoidable. All attempts to cover up the problem seem to fail. The idea of suicide seems to grow stronger. A study of people with body-dysmorphic disorder published in the *Journal of*

Clinical Psychiatry found that 78 percent of teens with this problem had contemplated suicide.

Another concern about plastic surgery on adolescents is that their bodies are still maturing. In addition to development that may occur in the late teens, growth charts indicate that the average young woman gains weight between the ages of eighteen and twenty-one, and that is likely to change her interest or need for breast augmentation and liposuction.

Why Reverse Pressure Works

Regardless of the naysayers, social pressure and personal anxieties will continue to motivate teenagers to have plastic surgery procedures. Requiring parental consent for patients under eighteen does not ensure informed consent, since research is lacking on long-term risks for many cosmetic procedures. Furthermore, today's parents are more likely to yield to the demands of their teens. Parents, of course, envision a bright and happy future for their children, and the knowledge of how competitive it is out there makes them push their wards to do well academically and socially. Thus, when their teenagers express the need for an aesthetic procedure to be successful in their environment, they usually face little resistance from their mothers and fathers. There are few obstacles in the way of teens who want to improve their appearance. It's simply going to happen.

Can Cosmetic Surgery Actually Be Good for Teens?

Let's begin with the social pressure adolescents face. Teens can be mean. Just ask **Jen**, **Jon**, and **Hannah**. For years, Jen endured taunts because of her nose size. Kids ridiculed her by saying she looked like a pelican and by calling her "butter face"—a code for "She's hot, but her face!"

Jon deliberately grew his hair out to hide ears that had branded him with the nickname "Dumbo." And Hannah's self-confidence flagged as she endured "horrifying" name-calling after developing DDD-size breasts as a teenager.

In a world where people of all ages increasingly turn to plastic surgery for reasons that are purely cosmetic—and in some cases, narcissistic—Jen, Jon, and Hannah said they opted to go under the knife as teenagers for different reasons. It wasn't something they did solely because of the relentless name-calling. It also had a whole lot to do with how they felt about themselves on a deeper level.

"My advice to teenagers is, don't have a nose job just 'cause you're worried about what other people say or think," said Jen, who had rhinoplasty done in the summer at age fifteen. "It all has to do with how you feel on the inside. And getting a nose job made me feel good inside and out."

But parents do need to be proactive. Some reputable plastic surgeons with teen patients recommend a series of at least four sessions with a therapist before moving forward with any procedures. The point of these sessions is to uncover underlying motives for wanting surgery, as well as to determine the emotional maturity of the patient.

Such precautionary steps are important because demand is on the rise. Prior to the COVID outbreak, 4 percent of all plastic surgeries were performed on teens. Nose and ear reshaping, acne and acne-scar treatment, breast augmentation, and breast reduction are popular procedures among teenage patients.

Generally speaking, plastic surgeons report that many teens want plastic surgery because they long to fit in with their friends, while many adults pursue plastic surgery because they want to stand out. But when a teen seeks out plastic surgery to correct a noticeable physical defect or to change a body part that's caused prolonged psychological distress, that can be a good thing, doctors say.

"It's no different than kids getting braces for crooked teeth," said Jen's plastic surgeon. Indeed, plastic surgery can be altogether positive in the right circumstances. In the cases of Jen, Jon, and Hannah, all of whom were featured in *People* magazine and interviewed on the *Today* show, the NBC network's chief medical doctor thought they had made responsible choices when they decided to have plastic surgery done at ages fifteen, seventeen, and nineteen.

For their parts, Jon, Hannah, and Jen all claim they have no regrets about their plastic surgeries. Jon's decision to have his ears pinned back made him feel good about cutting his hair to pursue his dream of becoming a firefighter. Hannah's breast reduction surgery gave her relief from pain and made it possible to maintain an active, athletic lifestyle. And Jen's nose job made her more confident and carefree.

"Jen is so happy now," said her mother, Jill. "I would say to parents...it's the greatest gift you could give to your child. What greater gift is confidence and to help them feel happy in who they are?"

Dr. Hardesty: Of course, teenagers often seek plastic surgery for a variety of understandable reasons, ranging from addressing a health need to fixing a feature that has made them susceptible to bullying. However, I agree with my medical body, the American Society of Plastic Surgeons, which emphasizes the importance of understanding a teen's motive for surgery and ensuring that every potential teenage patient undergoes a careful and extensive preoperative evaluation to ensure they are an appropriate candidate for their desired procedure.

Dr. Polakof: Let's face it. We aren't going to eliminate the siren call of social media, nor bullying or teenage insecurities. And frankly, many teens will resist having to undergo sessions with a psychologist to determine if they are mentally fit or are having an aesthetic procedure for the right reasons. I believe the responsibility for authorizing and monitoring a teenager's plastic surgery clearly lies in the hands of parents. It's completely acceptable to have several heart-to-heart talks with your children about their reasons for wanting surgery—and why not involve these kids in becoming responsible by sharing the financial burden? (Most cosmetic surgery isn't covered by insurance.)

Finally, parents should undertake the research we have outlined in this book as if they were having the aesthetic procedure themselves—thoroughly examining surgeon credentials, reviewing evidence of their work, asking the hard questions, and speaking to parents of other teenagers who have been patients.

CHAPTER 20

FUTURE OF PLASTIC SURGERY AND INNER BEAUTY

"The future is always beginning now."
—Mark Strand

The plastic surgery industry is already a massive money-generating enterprise. *Globe Newswire* reports that the plastic surgery market is likely to be worth almost sixty-seven billion dollars by 2026. It's a bright future, but what can we look forward to?

In the future, there will be fewer actual aesthetic surgeries, and nonsurgical procedures will largely dominate. There have been predictions that by 2050, less than 5 percent of all procedures will involve actual cosmetic surgery.

It will be possible to enlarge and enhance breasts, cheekbones, hip, abdominal, and pectoral zones by simply enriching the fat tissue taken from a person's body with stem cells and then reinjecting these into the needed areas. With stem-cell injections, hair loss (baldness) will be totally eliminated; drooping eyelids and sagging facial skin will be lifted and toned. Your own stem cell-enriched body fat will be transferred from your waist, thighs, or back, sculpting one area, and used as a natural filler to enhance breasts or butt for contouring and enhancement.

Aesthetic stem cell procedures are already in effect at some practices, but experts warn that much more science and development is required to achieve viable results and patient satisfaction. Additionally, it's been predicted that today's radiofrequency devices will be available just like blow dryers you use at home. In the future, you will be able to lift and tone your face or body as if you are doing your hair. Also, laser epilation (hair removal) devices will be as common as any domestic appliance.

And there are some actual predictions that, by 2050, the human being will no longer be the "human" we recognize today, but instead, a prototype of a biomechanical creature called a cyborg (cybernetic organism).

It's possible that, as we age, or are severely injured, a portion of our body will be artificial thanks to cardiac pacemakers, insulin pumps, metal joints, bone prostheses, artificial hearts, eyes, kidneys, ears, and noses, along with prosthetic arms and legs. Acne and pimples will vanish, and a multitude of body infections will be prevented by the vaccines discovered. Some say even our clothes will be nanotechnology products and thus will enable us to better adapt to the environmental conditions by not only protecting our body against all kinds of bacteria, but also adjusting the body temperature and moisture. They will help us to live a healthier life by adjusting our heartbeat, blood pressure, blood sugar, and hormones through state-of-the-art chips embedded in them.

Sleep, which is essential for beauty and a long life, will be regulated by a headpiece. Similarly, hunger and thirst will be regulated by these electronic devices on our heads, and it will be easier for us to maintain our ideal weight.

By 2050, people will not ask each other if they had an aesthetic surgery; instead, they will ask why they did not. It is normal that everyone wants to look beautiful in a society where all the bad TV and cinema characters are ugly. Certainly, in the near coming years, there will be great advances in medicine. Many surgical operations will be performed by microscopic (nanotechnology) devices or robots inserted into the body. For instance, a microscopic device inserted under the facial skin is predicted to be able to move around like a bulldozer or a scraper and correct the flaws, wrinkles, and sagging internally.

Incidentally, when recalling flying humans in the 1488 drawings of Leonardo da Vinci, one can only wonder if we will be able to give bird wings to human beings as a result of advanced gene technology.

In South Korea, Some of the Future Is Here Now

South Korea, particularly Seoul, is known as the plastic surgery capital of the world. The country is booming with plastic surgery businesses over recent years. Their new, enhanced technology, budget-friendliness, and tourism benefits have contributed to their worldwide ranking.

As for the culture around plastic surgery, the types of surgeries done in South Korea and the United States are representative of their societies. In both countries, people get surgery for the purpose of imitating their favorite celebrities and following new beauty standards. For instance, in America, when women see Kim Kardashian with enhanced features, a trim waistline, and a prominent butt, many want the same. When South Korean women see their favorite idols or actresses having ethereal features, they're ready to get that same look.

But when it comes to the value of surgery, that is where the countries differ. In the US, plastic surgery is often criticized and judged harshly, while cosmetic surgery is positive in South Korea. It is known to increase confidence and self-esteem, to feel and help become one's best version of themselves.

South Korean advances in technology have had a huge impact on the plastic surgery industry. With Korean cosmetic surgery, the rapid change in technology has given doctors the chance to progress in the way they perform procedures. Korean plastic surgeons actually have a greater gamut of noninvasive treatments than surgeons in the United States.

One example is the Gangnam-style surgery, located in Gangnam, which uses game-changing stem cell treatments to improve the look of the skin. Another modality is a machine which can treat skin problems without a need to cut into the skin. It is expected these unique procedures will come to the US in the future.

The most common plastic surgeries done in Seoul are double eyelid, jaw reduction, and chin reshaping. But with the addition of newly developed technology, the rise of minimal and noninvasive surgeries has begun to escalate over the past few years. Having easier access, more South Korean women can obtain a wide variety of noninvasive procedures in addition to Botox, fillers, and lifting. With medical improvements in these specific surgeries, this also means there are fewer side effects, and it is cheaper. These cosmetic surgeries are already in high demand in the US, but the difference between the two countries is the price. The cost of plastic surgery in South Korea is very competitive compared to some of the top Western countries offering a similar set of procedures. Flaunting the highest number of plastic surgeries performed on a global scale, South Korea is also recognized as the "plastic surgery capital" due to its experienced surgeons, advanced medical facilities, and satisfied patients.

What this means for plastic surgery in the US is that ultimately, cosmetic surgery will become more affordable. Plastic surgeons will need to compete against growing medical tourism, particularly in counties such as South Korea, where cosmetic surgery is safe and somewhat technologically advanced.

A New Era of Transparency Around Plastic Surgery

Marc Jacobs is well known as an American fashion designer renowned for his sartorial interpretations of trends in pop culture, perhaps most notably his "grunge" collection. Recently, he underwent a newer facelift procedure using the advanced deep plane technique which lifts only under the muscle layer, leaving the skin attached to the muscle layers to steer clear of tightness. This has shown to result in a smoother, softer lifted look.

The unusual aspect of Marc's surgical experience is that, while his 1.6 million followers are accustomed to seeing him share the ins and outs of his daily life on Instagram, there's something quite extraordinary about someone of Jacobs' stature pulling back the curtains so widely on their plastic surgery.

In order to do what he could to help shift societal attitudes and shed the stigma around plastic surgery, Marc actually chronicled his entire facelift experience in multiple posts on Instagram. And he was happy to help educate curious parties on the recovery and results of the latest cutting-edge procedures.

In one of his comments, Jacobs candidly discussed his postoperative recovery. "I love the results. I'm very happy. I'm still in the process of going to this hyperbaric oxygen chamber every day for a couple of hours, which is supposed to help with healing. There was some discomfort after the surgery where I took painkillers. I made sure I had a nurse who monitored those painkillers so that I wouldn't abuse them because I do have a problem with addiction, so I was very transparent with my people."

Marc's concluding comments are also extremely candid. "I'm fifty-eight years old. I don't think I look bad for fifty-eight years old. I didn't feel like I *had* to do this, but I feel like all of these conversations around aging or around plastic surgery are just like any other conversations to me. The problem comes with the shame around them. And I don't want to live my life with shame, you know? I find the way I do that is by being open, transparent, and honest about things. Yes, I'm vain. I find there is no shame in being vain. I find there's no shame in wanting attention. I find there's no shame in getting dressed up and showing off a look."

Fortunately, the celebrity taboo about admitting to having aesthetic plastic surgery is slowly lifting. Celebrities such as Kaley Cuoco, Cardi B, and Jana Kramer have been as admirably vocal as Marc Jacobs about their cosmetic tweaks. And lately, more name personalities are seeing the value in educating others as well.

The Future of Inner Beauty

Fortunately, society appears to be on a path of awareness that, in addition to physical attractiveness, we should look more closely at the beauty inside a person. In fact, we believe more and more people are beginning to realize inner beauty is a far more important asset—and fortunately, plastic surgery can help bring it to the surface.

A wise surgeon made the following comment:

> One question I wish I was asked more often is how to achieve and nurture inner beauty. We can achieve and nurture true beauty from the inside out by caring for ourselves, surrendering more often, and being gentle with ourselves under stress. The results of this inner beauty regimen are even more meaningful than a glowing face or reduced scarring or other signs we use to measure outer beauty. While skin will eventually age, our inner self only grows in wisdom and loveliness all the time.

Inner beauty is who you are, not what you look like. Inner beauty is more than skin deep, and it is not in the eye of the beholder. The great news about inner beauty is that you get to decide what "beautiful" means to you. It's worth taking the time to discuss what inner beauty is not. It doesn't look like judging other people, plastic surgery, or other external beauty efforts, or pushing yourself to fit unrealistic standards. Inner beauty means being loving to yourself, others, and the world around you. While looks may fade over time, inner peace and self-confidence grow more dazzling each year you practice them. When you take the time to care for your inner beauty, you're making an investment that will follow you for the rest of your life.

Real beauty is about becoming a person you're proud of—one who's gentle with herself and sets her own standards. The characteristics of inner beauty include being kind, loving yourself, maintaining positive self-esteem, and being at peace with the world.

When your beauty doesn't depend on simply your haircut or a new outfit, it becomes a gift you can give to others. True beauty makes you stronger, a better person, more honest, and the best version of yourself.

Dr. Hardesty: People with inner beauty are loving to others and themselves. However, many times, the way we discuss our bodies is anything but kind. In order to develop more self-love, it might be beneficial to change the language we use about our body. Your words have an impact on your body image and overall well-being.

It might be helpful to start with gratitude. Write out a list of all the reasons you're thankful for your body: how it helps you go places, or how your fingers let you type, or how it's created life in the form of children, art, or creative expression.

The more we focus on the positive aspects of the body we have, the less at war we will feel with it each day. Body shaming is thrown at us daily, but it's our choice to discard those superficial impressions and choose to acknowledge what is beautiful about ourselves.

Dr. Polakof: The latest statistics reveal that women constitute 92 percent of all aesthetic plastic surgery procedures. Thus, it's time for more sensitive and knowledgeable plastic surgeons to step up and take the pulse of true female patient interests. It's time to understand the need to place more emphasis upon inner beauty.

A woman's inner beauty needs to always be evident on the outside, and a plastic surgeon can and should strive to make this a reality. Sensitivity, integrity, honesty, and caring values are some of the precious traits that escalate a woman beyond physical attractiveness.

No matter what the situation or circumstances, a woman who possesses inner beauty will conduct herself in a manner that makes others take notice. The importance of quality life after COVID brings about many opportunities to fashion a woman's character for real inner beauty. This should be a joint effort between plastic surgeon and patient.

The End

ABOUT THE AUTHORS

Dr. James Polakof, PhD, is a medical consultant, nutritionist, and author dedicated to providing medical knowledge to patients. Having received his doctorate in nutrition, his engagement with thousands of people seeking medical advice led him to thirty-five years of medical marketing and sales. This allowed Dr. Polakof to create over seven hundred medical education programs for multiple medical fields, including plastic surgery. Besides his programs, he went on to write and host a mini-series with Erin O'Brien, produce two award-winning documentaries, and create his sensational podcast, *Discovering New Horizons*. Dr. Polakof currently lives in Pinehurst, North Carolina.

Dr. Robert Hardesty is a plastic surgeon and medical director known for over ten thousand operations in his thirty-year career. Receiving his education at the University of Pittsburgh and Washington University in St. Louis, he started the first integrated training program for future cosmetic surgeons at his alma mater, Loma Linda University, School of Medicine. Dr. Hardesty then went on to perform many successful plastic surgeries with high patient satisfaction before opening his medical spa, Imagine Plastic Surgery, in 2003. *The Real You, Only Better* will be his debut book. Former accolades include the presidency of the California Society of Plastic Surgery and the chairman of the Plastic Surgery Research Council. Dr. Hardesty continues leading his team at their surgery clinic in San Bernardino, California.

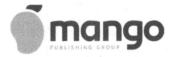

Mango Publishing, established in 2014, publishes an eclectic list of books by diverse authors—both new and established voices—on topics ranging from business, personal growth, women's empowerment, LGBTQ studies, health, and spirituality to history, popular culture, time management, decluttering, lifestyle, mental wellness, aging, and sustainable living. We were named 2019 *and* 2020's #1 fastest growing independent publisher by *Publishers Weekly.* Our success is driven by our main goal, which is to publish high-quality books that will entertain readers as well as make a positive difference in their lives.

Our readers are our most important resource; we value your input, suggestions, and ideas. We'd love to hear from you—after all, we are publishing books for you!

Please stay in touch with us and follow us at:

Facebook: Mango Publishing
Twitter: @MangoPublishing
Instagram: @MangoPublishing
LinkedIn: Mango Publishing
Pinterest: Mango Publishing
Newsletter: mangopublishinggroup.com/newsletter

Join us on Mango's journey to reinvent publishing, one book at a time.